CW00765457

Life After Birth

A guide to prepare, support and nourish
you through motherhood

Jessica Prescott and Vaughne Geary of Mama Goodness

For the mamas.

This book was created on the stolen land of the Wurundjeri People. We pay our respects
to Elders past and present, and acknowledge the deep connection Aboriginal and Torres Strait
Islander Peoples have with the land on which we live, work and create.

Hardie Grant

BOOKS

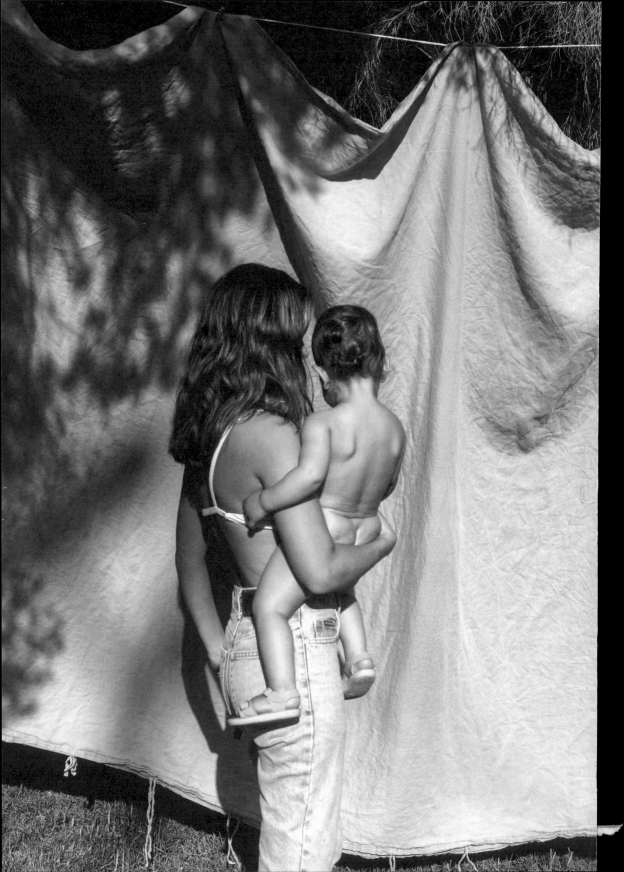

MEDICAL DISCLAIMER

This book is not intended as a medical reference and the statements and practices in this book do not take into account the health, medical, physical, psychological or emotional status of the reader. It should therefore not be used as a replacement for diagnosis and treatment of any condition, medical or otherwise.

This book is intended to share helpful and scientifically accurate information on the subjects discussed; however, the authors and publisher are not medical professionals and, as such, recommend seeking out any diagnosis and treatment of any condition with a qualified healthcare practitioner.

The reader should consider their own individual circumstances before acting on or using any of the information or advice shared in this book.

The author and publisher accept no liability for any consequences related to the following of advice in this book, or the following of advice on any of the resources shared in it.

With gratitude.

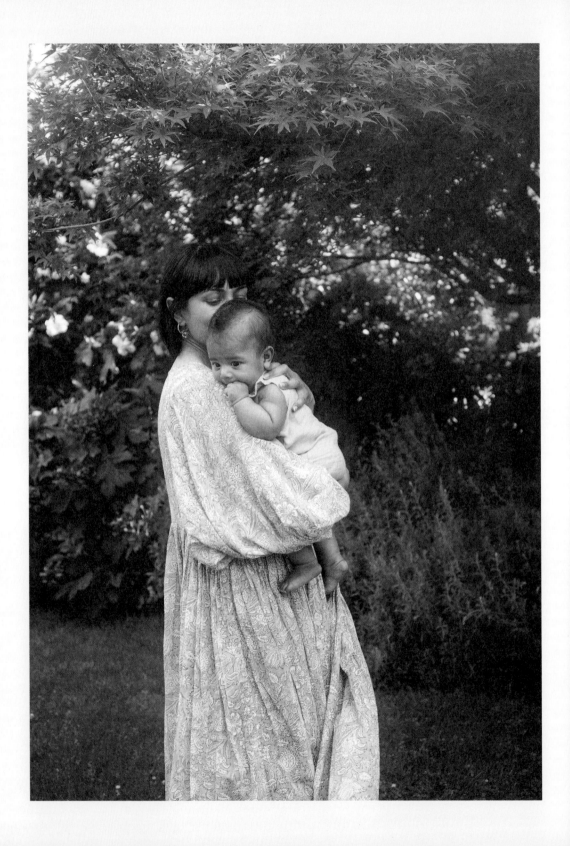

Contents

INTRODUCTION

We are quite possibly the first ever society to bear so little reverence to something as momentous as childbirth. The increasing commodification of motherhood has us more focused on how bringing a baby home *looks* than how it feels, with emotional support and nourishing meals being replaced by the Pinterest nursery, the perfect pram and matching beige outfits.

There is an inordinate amount of pressure for birthing people to 'bounce back' – not only to their pre-baby weight, but also to their pre-baby way of living, despite everything their mind, body and spirit has gone through in the growing and birthing of a baby. On top of this, there is very little cultural support or understanding of JUST HOW F*CKING HARD IT IS to raise a family.

Nothing is the same. How can it be, when our entire centre of gravity has shifted so immensely? Yet we routinely attend our six-week postpartum check-up to be told by a doctor that we are (or aren't) healed enough to resume intercourse, asked whether we want any kind of contraception and sent on our merry way.

The ripple effect of the gaping wide hole in postpartum care has people stumbling through parenthood, often feeling under-resourced, exhausted, depleted, anxious and depressed. It puts pressure on relationships, and strain on the social and economic infrastructures we belong to.

But all is not lost. As we write this, there is a strong undercurrent – one that is challenging bounce-back culture and honouring the cataclysmic transition that follows the birth of a child. A movement that centres the mother, rather than just the baby, because while of course the baby is of utmost importance, the wellbeing of every family constellation is dependent on the wellbeing of the mother they orbit.

When we combine ancient wisdom with the most current neurological, physiological and nutritional research, we learn how to use the weeks after birth as a time for respite, recovery and rejuvenation, which sets us up to thrive through the months and years that follow.

We have witnessed firsthand how mothers and communities thrive when proper care is given. In this book we share some of the tips and tools we have picked up over the past decade or so, with our combined experience as postpartum doulas, as well as Jess being a mother and Vaughne being a naturopath and nutritionist.

In these pages we cover everything from how to prepare during pregnancy, what foods to fill your pantry with and what conversations to have with loved ones as you prepare for this momentous inner work, to breastfeeding, what to truly expect when you bring your baby home, postpartum nutrition and herbal support, sex after baby, parenting tips and so much more. It's the postpartum bible that every birthing person needs.

Our aim with this book is to provide guidance and support for all people on the wide and diverse spectrum of motherhood, and shift the narrative to a more realistic one. We want people to feel safe admitting they aren't coping, and we want to normalise the challenges that parents of small humans go through, so that others know how to help. We want help to become the norm, and not the thing people seek out only when they are at rock bottom.

While no book can ever truly prepare you, we hope to provide you with an invaluable guide that enables you to step into this new chapter of life with knowledge, power, grace and ease, even when you're covered in shit. We want you to feel resourced, nourished and empowered, so you can find magic in the mundane, and celebrate all the big, little and hilarious moments you are gifted by your children every day.

It's time to rally our entire extended community to think differently about mothers and birthing people, and how to better support them. This is our contribution.

'As women, we recognise the qualities of courage, love and surrender it takes to go through childbirth. After each birth we are changed in a momentous way, on all levels, and it takes these same qualities to recognise our vulnerability and allow ourselves to heal and enter motherhood.

To do the best for ourselves does not mean following a rigid set of rules after childbirth. Our own Golden Month is essentially a question of understanding what is happening in the postpartum, recognising the wisdom of our traditions and listening inward to the messages of our bodies – then putting these pieces of knowledge together, in the context of being held by family and community.'

JENNY ALLISON, *GOLDEN MONTH,*
BEATNIK PUBLISHING (REVISED EDITION 2021)

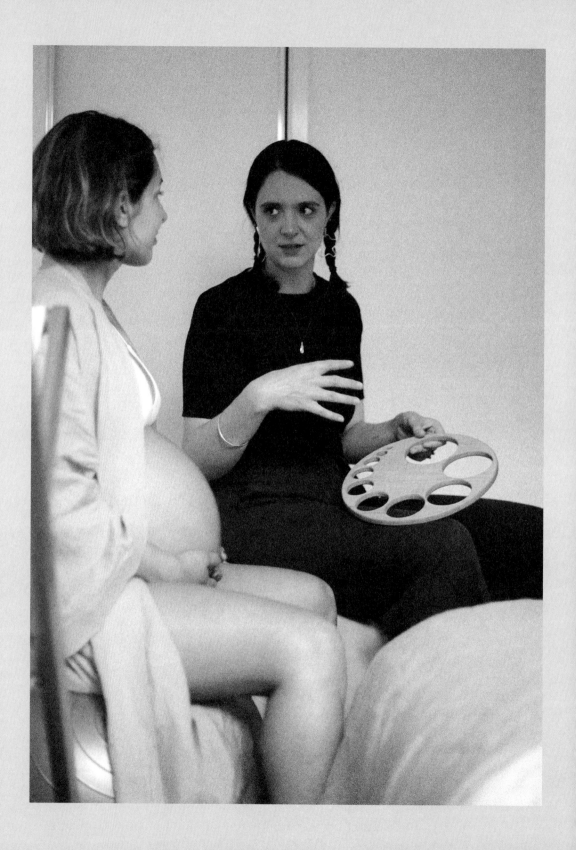

WHAT IS A DOULA AND WHAT DO THEY DO?

A doula is a space holder for the most epic transformations of the human experience.

While society is becoming aware of the existence and role of birth doulas, many don't realise that doulas also exist for postpartum support, abortion or miscarriage support and death support.

The idea behind inviting a doula into your postpartum or birth space is ancient and seen across many cultures around the world. Having someone you trust by your side to hold space while you unravel, listen without judgement, care for you, feed you healing and nourishing food, and educate you on your options for the journey ahead, has the ability to empower you during the most tender and vulnerable time of your life.

A doula's offerings are varied and incredibly individual, with many of them having a background in counselling, midwifery, naturopathy, massage, and all kinds of other incredible care work. How their support looks will differ from client to client, with their visits tailored to the individual needs of the families they are supporting.

During pregnancy, your doula will connect and bond with you and your partner, discuss and deconstruct your personal and socio-cultural beliefs surrounding birth, help you to create preferences for your birth and postpartum experience, debrief appointments you've had with other care providers, and help you to physically and emotionally prepare for labour and birth. When you are in labour, they will join you at home or in the hospital to guide you through the momentous journey of birthing your baby.

During the postpartum, doulas commonly visit you in the comfort of your own home, making their care incredibly holistic, humble and intimate. They provide evidence-based knowledge and practical, hands-on support for you and your baby, as well as a safe space to debrief not only your birth, but the nitty-gritty of early parenthood and all the highs and lows that come with it. They are also there to provide resources in areas such as baby care, breastfeeding, mental health support and community building, so that you feel fully supported to make choices that feel intuitively right for you and your family.

We are both doulas, and we started Mama Goodness because we are deeply passionate about making sure that mums and birthing people receive the care that they so greatly deserve. We hope that in writing this book, we are able to extend our care to the far corners of the globe, so that even if we aren't with you in person, we can support you as you step across the sacred threshold of parenthood.

THE POSTPARTUM PILLARS

Most postpartum practitioners believe that there are six foundational pillars that are essential for optimal emotional, physical and spiritual wellbeing during the fourth trimester.

1
Rest

From 'cuarentena' in Mexico to 'confinement' in China, women in the family and village have always banded together to ensure the new mother gets the rest she needs following the momentous feat of childbirth. We can take heed of these traditions from cultures that understand the importance of rest and step in to carry out essential household tasks, care for other children, ensure the new mother is fed nourishing meals and is getting enough sleep. This leaves the mother with just one focus: taking care of and bonding with her baby. On a physiological level, rest is important for helping the body to heal, and it supports the nervous system and hormones to recalibrate and regulate after pregnancy and birth. This creates a vital window of opportunity to build and restore health reserves, and optimise the new mother's wellbeing for years to come.

2
Nourishment

From a naturopathic lens, and that of many other cultures that innately tend to mothers in their postpartum, food is considered medicine. It provides macro- and micronutrients that our body utilises for energy, metabolic regulation, hormone production and reproductive health, amongst so many other functions. After birth, the body is in a state of flux and repair, which requires essential nutritional building blocks to recover and ensure that both mother and baby are given a chance to thrive. Without the therapeutic benefits of quality food during postpartum, mothers can experience delayed healing and vulnerability to various ailments that can affect them for years to come. The warmth and nourishment of complex carbohydrates, healthy fats and protein, fibrous fruits and vegetables, hydration and therapeutic herbs and spices offers a multitude of benefits for physical and mental recovery, and the future health of a mother.

3
Warmth

In cultures around the world there is a strong emphasis on staying warm after giving birth, as it is understood that regardless of whether you have a vaginal or caesarean birth, blood loss results in a reduction of circulation and body temperature. Staying warm in the early postpartum encourages the production of oxytocin and the contraction of the uterus to its pre-pregnancy size, thus reducing blood loss and promoting circulation and milk production. Not only this, but it is thought that in order to balance the intense, outward and opening energy of birth, we should focus on keeping our womb space and body warm so that the mother can turn inward, reflect, rest and recover. Bringing warmth into your postpartum may look like comfy socks, warm baths, pelvic steaming, and consuming plenty of warm drinks and meals cooked with thermogenic spices.

4
Physical Touch

Studies have shown just how essential touch is for both humans and animals in their ability to survive from the moment they are born. In the days and weeks after birth, a mother's body undergoes immense changes: physically, emotionally and hormonally. Blood volume and fluid carried during pregnancy are reducing, organs and structural bones, muscles and ligaments are returning to their optimal position, and mothers are often very tender as they navigate their new body and emotions. The health benefits of bodywork such as massage and osteopathy, as well as the simple embrace of another, have been found to calm the nervous system, while lowering blood pressure and stress hormones. Consensual physical touch, whether from a partner, friend or therapist, activates the vagus nerve, which is intimately involved in the release of the 'love hormone', oxytocin. Many cultures around the world nurture new mothers with bodywork, such as *abhyanga* massage in India, and 'Closing the Bones' ceremonies in Mexico.

5
Community

A new parent cannot thrive without the helping hands of those who they trust and confide in the most. Having a truly nourished and nurtured postpartum takes time, effort and dedication. In stark contrast to cultures who practise postpartum confinement with the support of generations of women, Western society has bred generations of people who believe that individuality is best and asking for help has come to mean failure when, in fact, it is what humans need most. Because many of us live far away from our families and often don't even know our neighbours, it is up to us to build our own village. Many hands make light work, and in the early postpartum this may look like the support of a doula, midwife or friends and family cooking a meal train. Once you leave your postpartum cocoon and your child grows older, this will open up to include the wide and diverse community of people you meet through parenthood.

6
Nature

We live in a world that is increasingly high-tech, and everything from the way we work to the way we socialise causes us to look down at gadgets and remain indoors, rather than looking up into nature and the beauty that surrounds us. Once you have children, life all of a sudden requires a slower pace and you may find yourself noticing the parallels between parenthood and nature. There is so much to learn from the change of seasons, both outside your window and in your new life as a mother. Everything unfolds within its own unique timeline and neither nature, nor children, can be rushed. Plants, used in culinary or medicinal form are also incredibly therapeutic and provide essential nutrients and healing properties for parents and children alike. Science is continuously proving how strong our affinity for nature is, and you can reconnect to it in an abundance of simple ways, such as drinking herbal tea, filling your home with plants or visiting your favourite park, creek, lake or beach.

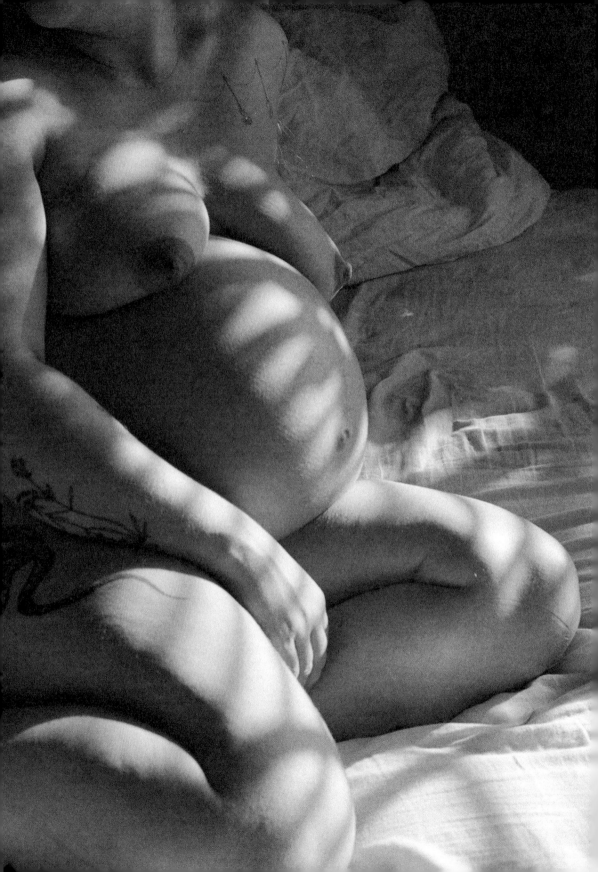

PREPARING FOR

CHAPTER ONE

YOUR POSTPARTUM

'The ancient wisdom of Ayurveda explains that the first 42 days after birth is a "Kayakalpa", a sacred window of time where a person has an opportunity for incredible healing at an accelerated pace. This is a unique window that one experiences only a few times during their life. When proper care is given during this window, the effects of that care will last the person far into the future. When mothers and birthing people are given conscious love and care with attention to their specific needs, we are not only serving that person, but their family, our communities and the world.' – Christine Devlin Eck

When your baby is earthside and you embark on the journey of becoming a parent, it rarely looks the same or comes as easily as you imagined it would. There is so much change and uncertainty in those blurry newborn days, and the difference in how your fourth trimester will shape you lies in the amount of mental and physical preparation and support you have in place. Knowing what to expect, surrounding yourself with wise women and helping hands, and arming yourself with the tools and education you need to be able to look after yourself, can make your postpartum one of the most restful and empowering times of your life.

While writing this book, we did a social media call out for people's advice about motherhood – we wanted to make sure we left no stone unturned, and no topic untouched. The overwhelming response was – plan for your postpartum. While birth prep is incredibly important, many people went blindly into their postpartum and said if they could do it again, they would have planned more, or at least gathered an awareness about what to expect afterwards, instead of focusing solely on the birth.

'Preparing for your birth but not your postpartum is like preparing for your wedding but not your marriage.'

NAOMI CHRISOULAKIS

Throughout this chapter there are questions and journal prompts to help you reflect as you prepare for your fourth trimester and new life as a mother. Grab yourself, a blank journal, and commit to writing from a place of total honesty.

YOUR BRAIN

If you are pregnant while reading this, you have no doubt already noticed changes in your brain. Pregnancy can make you more emotional, unbelievably tired, and sensitive (to smells, energy, everything), and it's no wonder when you consider the biological processes that are occurring. Not only are your organs shifting and belly expanding to make way for a new life growing inside you, but your brain is also under the influence of a strong cocktail of hormones (hello oestrogen, progesterone and oxytocin) and neurological changes that make growing, birthing and feeding that life possible.

As your pregnancy progresses, you may become forgetful – not only about where you put your keys or how to do simple algebra, but about passwords and PINs too. Society trivialises these changes, but, like the physical changes we undergo in pregnancy, they are part of our divine human design: a neurological fine-tuning that is priming us to protect our baby and be the best mothers we can be. After all, this is as important for the survival and wellbeing of our species as pregnancy and birth itself.

Expanding Belly, Shrinking Brain

While not nearly enough research has been done on the brain during pregnancy, what we do know is that pregnancy leads to a decrease in grey matter, or – a shrinking of the brain. This architectural reshape occurs with such consistency that an MRI scan is able to detect the changes in the brain of anyone who has ever given birth. It is thought that this decrease in grey matter leads to a sharpening of our social senses, increasing our ability to interpret non-verbal cues, thus making us more attuned to our baby's needs.

In addition, from pregnancy to the first two years of your baby's life, your brain's neuroplasticity increases, meaning it is able to create new pathways, making you more open to learning and change. As we attune to our baby's needs and become more sensitive to the world around us, we may find ourselves with increased empathy, emotional intelligence, resilience, ambition and efficiency, which could be why many women opt for a career change once they have children.

Dr Renee White says, 'While your overall brain size is significantly reduced, particular regions of your brain increase. From the moment of placental implantation, a mama's brain begins to modify crucial regions responsible for the "maternal circuitry", including modifications to reduce maternal stress, anxiety, fear and increase nesting and the protection of our babies. Throughout pregnancy, your brain is evolving and triaging cognitive functions in preparation for the birth of your child. Research shows that while there is a "fogginess" in the first few weeks postpartum, your brain is effectively levelling up from novice to expert in your new baby game. Never fear, the feelings are transient and give way to improved cognitive functions. Every time you are pregnant, your brain undergoes this process again, essentially levelling you up to genius.'

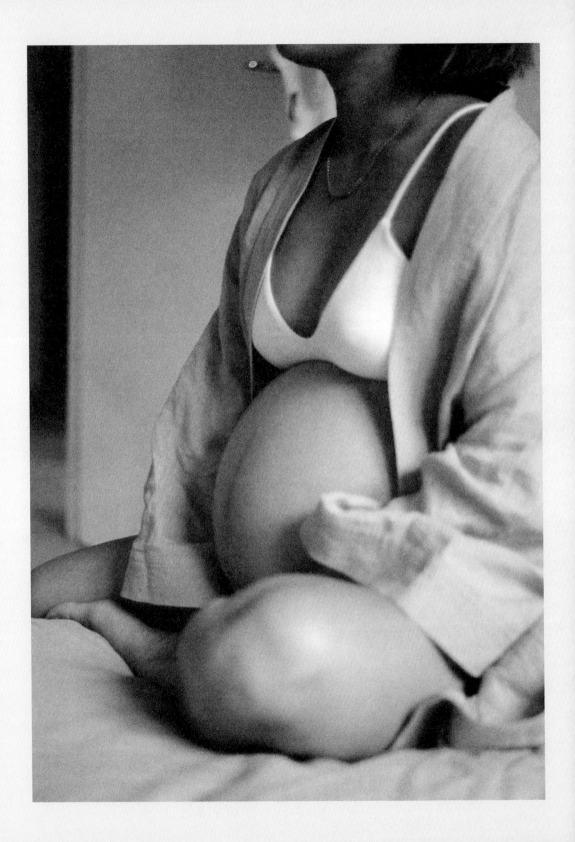

Oxytocin, the Love Hormone

The other major change that happens in our brains during pregnancy is the increase in both production of and reception to oxytocin, which is involved in attachment, bonding, mental health, milk ejection and uterine contractions. As well as facilitating the bonding process between mother and baby, it promotes feelings of wellness and has analgesic properties, making us less susceptible to pain.

Oxytocin is *the* postpartum hormone. It's what everyone wants to cultivate in their postpartum and it is the goal of every holistic birth and postpartum practitioner to 'keep the oxytocin flowing' once the baby is earthside, because of its importance in protecting the mother–baby dyad. The more we produce, the better we are at bonding with and caring for our babies. This promotes the production of oxytocin in their little bodies too, resulting in a more content baby who is better able to form positive attachments to their caregivers.

Cortisol, the Stress Hormone

Cortisol is a known oxytocin buster, meaning things such as stress, sleep deprivation, hunger, domestic tasks, a crying baby, and trauma all interfere with oxytocin production. While these things can't always be avoided, we can mitigate their impact by having oxytocin boosting tricks up our sleeve.

Oxytocin Boosters

While things like holding your baby, looking into their eyes, breastfeeding and skin-to-skin contact all promote oxytocin, it's good to have a list of boosters in mind. That way you'll know how to get your oxytocin flowing in times where you feel overwhelmed or out of sorts, or when you feel like you're wading through a minefield of nappies and sleepless nights.

What sparks joy in your soul and brings you contentment? There are no wrong answers. This isn't about what you *think* should be bringing you joy and contentment, but what truly does. If binge watching feel-good TV shows while your baby snoozes on your chest is what does it for you – great. If you prefer a cup of tea in the bath – also great. Other oxytocin boosters may include yoga, meditation, a light stretch, being outdoors in nature, filling your home with flowers, cuddling your partner or pet, eating your favourite food, listening to your favourite song or podcast, even some light cooking if that's what fills your cup.

Make a list and refer back to it when emotions are running high and you need to calm down or hit the reset button.

Skin-to-skin Care (SSC)

Skin-to-skin care (also known as kangaroo care) is one of the most profound oxytocin boosters of all, with many studies showing an increase in the oxytocin levels of both mother and baby during skin-to-skin contact. SSC involves placing your naked baby on your bare chest (they can be wearing a diaper), which stimulates the production of oxytocin while lowering cortisol. Mothers with higher oxytocin levels exhibit more attunement and responsiveness to their babies, thus strengthening the mother–baby dyad. It should be noted that this is applicable to both the birth parent and the non-gestational parent. Why are we telling you this now, before your baby is even here? So that you can prepare for the 'golden hour'.

Preparing for the 'Golden Hour'

The 'golden hour' is when you have uninterrupted skin-to-skin contact during the first hour of your baby's life. Babies tend to be very alert in the first hour following birth and may perform the breast crawl (see page 50) before nursing for the first time. Following this, they may be very sleepy as they rest and recover from the birth process. Allowing SSC to continue for as long as possible is ideal, as it helps to regulate a baby's temperature, breathing and blood sugar, after having only ever known life in a controlled environment. On an energetic level, observing the golden hour protects the shared energy between the birthing person and their baby, who are interconnected and interdependent.

While many hospitals around the world are routinely observing SSC in the first hour (at least) of the baby's life, we recommend confirming that this is supported by your healthcare provider, as well as including it into your 'birth preferences', to ensure that if possible, immediately after birth, your naked baby is placed on your bare chest.

Of course, there are going to be instances where this cannot happen, such as in the case of obstetric emergencies. If you do miss out on observing the 'golden hour', allowing as much SSC with your baby when it is safe and possible to do so still has innumerable benefits for both parents and baby.

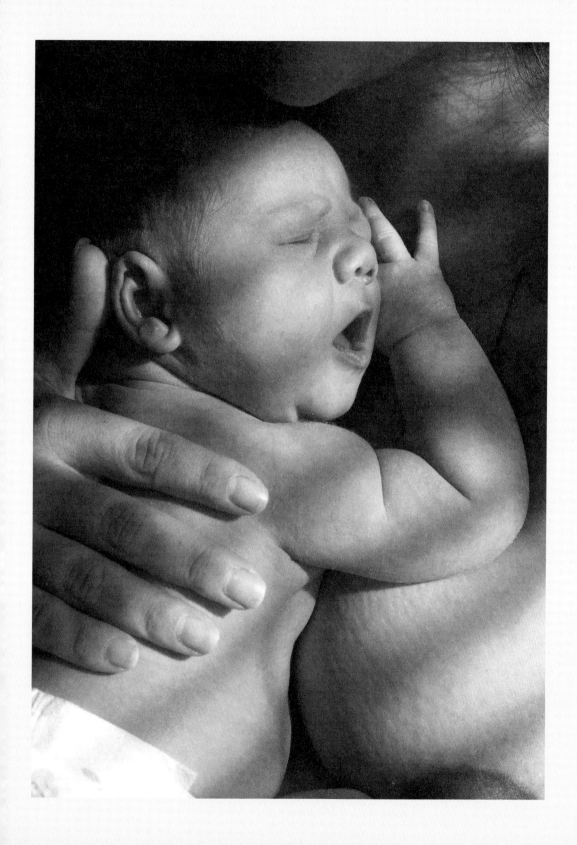

YOUR SELF

Matrescence

The term 'matrescence' was coined by anthropologist Dana Raphael to describe the journey from maiden to mother. It can be used to define *all* the changes – neurological, physical, emotional, hormonal, spiritual and social – that come with the growing and birthing of a baby. Similar in intensity to adolescence (which is the transition from childhood to adulthood), but with far less support and social understanding, matrescence is a rite of passage that often propels us into a journey of self-discovery that can be beautiful, painful and healing.

Not only do we find ourselves in a newfound state of vulnerability after we give birth, but with a burning desire to provide the best version of ourselves to our children and with this comes a new sense of identity that leaves us wondering where we belong in society. It is likened to a fracturing of the soul and it affects every fibre of our being, changing our relationship with the rest of the world, forever.

Like all great transitions in life, we need our periods of matrescence to be supported and validated by people who we love and trust. This is where your support network is vital – they can hold you through the changes, remind you that it's all normal, and guide you when you feel lost.

'Understanding that matrescence happens, that there is a reason why the transition to motherhood can feel so big, so intense, so earth shaking and soul stretching is powerful. But working WITH the changes, using this as an opportunity to reflect on your life, your beliefs, your values, your direction, the stories you carry about what it means to be a woman and mother will completely change your life.'

NIKKI McCAHON

Leaning Into Your Intuition

Learning to hear and trust your intuition while you're pregnant is one of the greatest tools you can have as a mother.

Intuition, also known as your 'sixth sense' or 'gut feeling', is an innate guiding force that has been relied on by our ancestors since time immemorial. Intuition is a protective mechanism that stems from our brain categorising every experience we've ever had as humans, and then guiding us with this knowledge in our day-to-day life. It is a *felt* sense, a *knowing* rather than logic.

Jane Hardwicke Collings says in her book *Ten Moons*, 'Perhaps this motherly intuition is the ongoing effect of the mother–baby connection, the energetic umbilical cord, so to speak. During pregnancy, our intuition sharpens just as our sense of smell does. Practice listening to your body and your feelings and you will sharpen your intuition.'

A good way to tune into your intuition while you are pregnant is to start letting your body make decisions for you. When presented with an idea – say for example, an invitation to a social event – tune into the initial reaction of your body. Does your body say yes or does your body say no? 'Yes' may be felt as excitement, calm, or relief, whereas 'No' may be felt as anxiety, apprehension or resistance. This initial response can be more trustworthy than our mind, which clouds our intuition with obligations, preconceptions and stories as part of its decision making process.

This may sound abstract, but you will find that there is an ease that comes with only saying 'yes' to things your body says 'yes' to. Listening to and trusting those feelings will pave the way for you to be more confident in your decisions not only as a parent, but in all aspects of your life. Learning how to trust your intuition is a way of protecting yourself from the constant streams of advice from family members, friends and other parents. While some of their advice can be helpful, it can also be conflicting, so it's beneficial to learn what feels right for you on a deeper level.

The Art of Surrender

While sometimes the word 'surrender' invokes a power dynamic, in parenting we like to define it as a softening and opening to change. Most things in motherhood are outside your control; learning to surrender makes this loss of control a lot easier to deal with.

On a practical level, being able to surrender to the monotony and logistics of parenthood is a vital step in regulating our nervous system and supporting our mental health. This may include not being able to tidy and vacuum because you are stuck under a clingy baby, or not making it out of the home when you thought you would (enter longer than expected naps, extended feeding sessions and poo explosions).

At times, the intense demands of parenthood can feel relentless. If you are able to let go and surrender to the present, you will be met not only with a feeling of ease, but space to recognise and lean into what works best for your unique mother–baby dyad. This fosters a trusting relationship between you and your baby and provides the potential for a new mindset that can make parenting easier and more enjoyable.

JOURNAL PROMPTS

1. Do you find it hard to relinquish control?
2. What would your partner say to this question? ;)
3. In what areas of your life can you let go a little (or a lot)?

Learning to Accept Help

Of all the self-work we are encouraging you to do, this can be the hardest. Control, shame, lack of worth, guilt and fear of rejection or being misunderstood come into play here, and it's no wonder when you look at the societal expectations of mothers. To a large degree, the Western world has lost touch with the notion of a 'village'. It takes work and courage to break down the barriers to accepting help, but it is essential, especially if you are parenting alone or far away from the support of close friends and family. Realising the value of being helped is an important step to receiving the care you deserve. If you struggle with this, remember that asking for and receiving help is a strength, not a weakness, and you are worthy of all help available – paid or unpaid.

Paid help may include hiring a doula, a cleaner or ordering prepared meals. Unpaid help might be accepting meals from your community or allowing friends to fold your laundry or walk your dog. Ideally, it helps to let go of the idea that you need to give something back in return. By doing this, you are creating space to heal, bond with your baby, and rest in a manner that will set you up to thrive in motherhood.

JOURNAL PROMPTS

1. Do you struggle to ask for help? If yes, why does it feel hard?
2. What are some ways you can ask for help?
3. In what areas of your postpartum can you imagine you'll need the most help?

Self Reflection and Identifying Triggers

Even if you had an idyllic childhood with seemingly perfect parents who will transition seamlessly into supportive grandparents, there may be foundational aspects of your upbringing that you hope to re-create, and some you would like to improve upon when you have your own family. Many of us recognise qualities in our own parents that we wish to embody and pass onto our own children, and others we wish to heal or leave behind.

In addition to that, most of us have past experiences that we would benefit from processing and making peace with. Until we do, our nervous system remains primed to respond to certain 'triggers'. Triggers often cause intense emotional reactions, and are linked to memory. They can be behaviours, smells, places or experiences and our responses to them can cause us to experience frustration, anger or rage, lash out, or even disassociate.

Using your time during pregnancy to identify your triggers, reflect on your past, do self-work and inner excavation, and have difficult or healing conversations will set the foundations for a supported transition into parenthood.

This may not be easy, but it is important for healing, and for ensuring our children don't have to take on our unhealed traumas. Seeking out professional help is often invaluable when reconciling your past, allowing you to feel self-acceptance and understanding, and helping you to develop emotional regulation tools.

JOURNAL PROMPTS

1. We all have triggers, what are yours?
2. How do you feel – emotionally and physically – when you are triggered?
3. Are you able to identify where these triggers stem from?

Emotional Regulation

Emotional regulation refers to the capacity to understand, monitor and regulate your emotional states and expressions, and the ability to calm yourself down and recalibrate when your nervous system is out of whack. It is an awareness that you are in control of your reactions to stressors and triggers from the outside world. The nervous system is an intricate operating system, which many humans cannot easily control in times of stress, because when our stress receptors are triggered, we have difficulty in concentrating, thinking clearly and being conscious of the needs of people around us.

For many of us, emotional regulation is something we learn as adults, because emotional regulation tools were not modelled to us as children (our parents didn't have these tools, because their parents didn't have these tools, and so on). If we grew up in homes where our parent figures responded to big emotions by exploding or withdrawing, this is likely how we respond to big emotions too. For some, a bowl of cereal accidentally falling on the floor may have sent their parents into an explosive rant and for others it may have been laughed off and cleaned up without any drama.

It is therefore important to find tools that help you manage your emotions and behaviours, as a key to teaching your children how to manage theirs. Much like flight attendants ask you to put your oxygen mask on before helping others, you will function much more effectively as a parent when you learn to regulate your own emotions before raising another human who will live and learn under your influential wing.

We all dream of having a calm baby, but babies are not born with innate regulation tools; they must learn them from us and they do this through co-regulation. Your baby will tune into your nervous system, paying attention to your heart rate, breathing, tone of voice, facial expressions and body language.

Learning to regulate your emotions is one of the greatest gifts you will ever give your children, because the way we respond to stress and conflict – including the inevitable meltdowns that even the most angelic of children will have – is the way your children will respond to stress and conflict for the rest of their lives.

How to Practise Emotional Regulation

TAKE A DEEP BREATH

When you're met with a challenging or triggering situation and feel that you're about to react, taking a deep breath can help to create space between yourself and the event that's unfolding. On a physical level, breath is your best friend, as it helps to slow your heart rate, regulate your nervous system and promote feelings of calm.

IDENTIFY WHAT YOU'RE FEELING

Take a moment to turn inward and notice the physical sensations in your body. Does your chest feel tight? Is there tension in your shoulders? Do you feel like crying? Or exploding? By tuning into these physical sensations, this again creates space between the trigger and your reaction, while allowing you to identify the emotions you are feeling.

NAME YOUR EMOTIONS

Once you have created space to identify the physical sensations in your body, you will have the mental clarity to identify and name your emotions. Do you feel rage? Fear? Shame? Disappointment? Often, there are multiple emotions hiding beneath the most prevalent one. When you are able to name them, this can help you make sense of what is happening and why you're reacting, while also helping you to communicate your emotions with others.

PAUSE AND REFLECT

As you become better at pausing, breathing and recognising your reactions to the world around you, you will notice just how normal it is to experience a multitude of emotions on any given day. With time and practise, you will become better at regulating your emotions and less reactive to every big and little thing that challenges or triggers you.

GIVE YOURSELF GRACE

You won't always get it right – no one does! Be patient, know that you are trying, and be so very proud of your incredible efforts. This is the work that positively impacts and rewrites the relationship you have with yourself and the people around you.

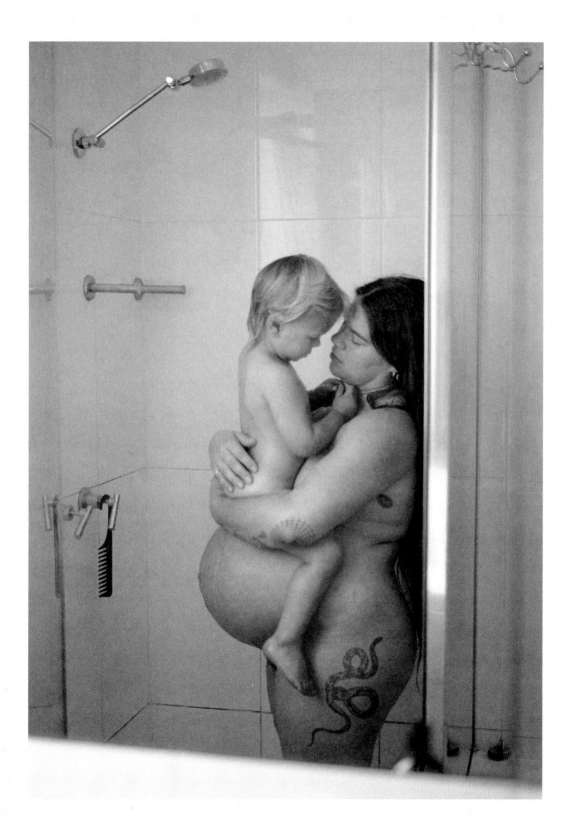

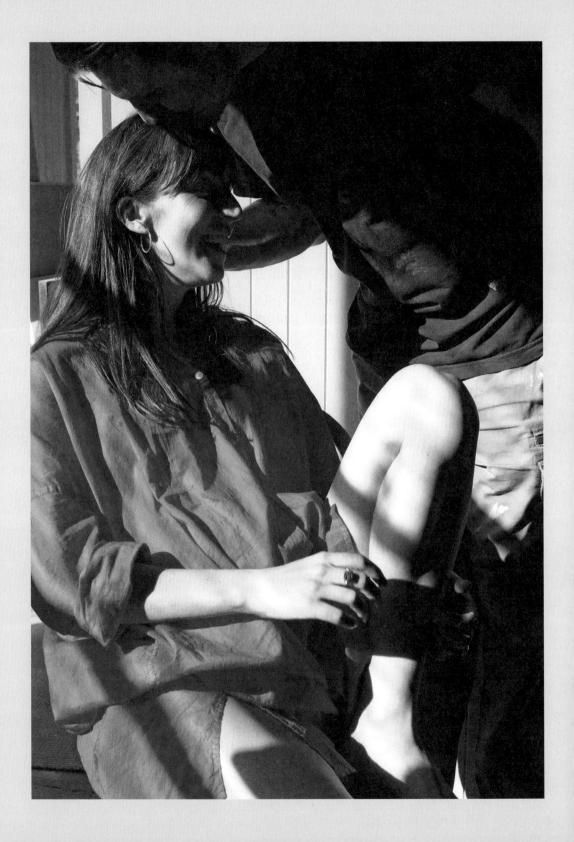

YOUR RELATIONSHIPS

Your Partner

If you are having a baby with a partner, no matter how rock-solid your relationship is, parenthood will test it beyond your wildest imagination. While it is one of the greatest joys of the human experience, it is also one of the biggest stressors on any relationship. It's not surprising when you consider the sleep deprivation, hormonal changes, and the fact that every waking moment is now focused on a tiny human who relies on you for their survival.

Up until now it's been just the two of you, and welcoming a baby will add a whole other dimension to the dynamics of your relationship. Discussing expectations of parenthood and of each other before your baby arrives is vital for keeping the foundations strong.

How will you ensure that you are both taking care of yourselves mentally and physically? And when will you find time to reconnect? Staying connected amidst the blur of milk and nappies will be the glue that sticks you together during this exhausting time.

Even the most unified partnership needs love and attention. It is important for both of you to find time each day to check in and ensure you feel seen and supported. Not communicating will cause things to fester, and exhaustion can amplify our reactions to things that bother us. Try to be gentle and understand that you are undergoing a huge transition and this can be a lonely and overwhelming time for partners.

Planning how you will manage your needs and having honest conversations about your expectations will help prevent unnecessary conflicts. Not only do you need to discuss emotional changes, but also practical ones. How will you manage finances? Who will vacuum the house and unpack the dishwasher? Who will do most of the cooking? It's wise to delegate tasks and is important for mothers to REST in the early weeks of the postpartum. Learning to be okay with things not being done 'your way' or as frequently and thoroughly as you would like, can be the difference between a calm and cooperative partnership and one that is fraught with tension.

One of the greatest tools that we've learnt during psychotherapy sessions is the concept of 'The Story in My Head'. Many conflicts happen due to miscommunication and we often create stories about our partner's intentions that are different from reality. When you're filled with sadness, rage or disbelief at something your partner has said or done (or not done), the ability to say 'the story in my head is ...' opens up communication and can help others see things from your perspective without feeling wrongly accused or attacked. It has saved both of us from major conflicts in our relationships.

CONVERSATION PROMPTS

1. When it comes to practising self-care as individuals, what are the non-negotiables for you and your partner?
2. What makes you feel connected as a couple?
3. What are you happy to let slide in your immediate postpartum?

Your Children

If you are pregnant with your second child, you've no doubt heard the saying 'your love doesn't halve, it doubles'. It can be difficult to imagine loving another baby as much as you love your firstborn, and you may find yourself fraught with guilt and worrying about how your other child/ren will transition into their role as sibling. If you had a relatively easy time with your first baby, it can be hard to imagine it being any different with your second, however the addition of a new family member is bound to bring up big emotions at some point.

Just as all adults differ in their emotional needs and reactions to change, so do children. Some will take it in their stride, loving on their new sibling like it is their own baby, while others may ignore the tiny elephant in the room or even revert to a baby-like version of themselves.

It's not unusual to experience grief as your relationship with your firstborn changes. Newborns have very different needs to their older siblings and you can't tend to them all at once. You are giving your child the gift of a sibling, and there is no relationship in their life that will be the same as this one. Keeping this in mind can help in the moments of guilt and uncertainty, and remember – they are gaining more in a sibling than they are losing in you as a mother. That being said, preparing your firstborn using some of the tips below can help ease their transition as your family grows.

- Plan at least 10 minutes of connection with your older children every day. Read them a book in bed while your partner holds the baby, play or take a bath together, or chat and cuddle with them. Allow them to lead if possible, offering them whatever you have the capacity for. The key here is that it's one-on-one time with no phones, babies or other interruptions.
- Maintain consistent connection during important times of the day such as mealtimes or bedtime, as well as creating connectivity with inside jokes, special phrases and loving touch where you can.
- Create a special basket of toys or a 'treasure box' for your child to play with when you need them to be quietly entertained while you tend to the needs of your baby. See our tips about sensory tubs on page 162.
- Talk about the baby often and encourage your firstborn to talk to the baby in your belly.
- Involve them in every aspect, including what you're going to name the new baby, setting up the baby's room or shopping for clothes and nappies. After the baby is born, continue inviting them to do small things to make them feel helpful and important, such as passing you a nappy.
- Purchase a toy you know your firstborn really wants and give it to them once the baby arrives as a gift to say 'thank you for being my big sibling'. Allow your older child to reciprocate by taking them shopping to pick out a 'birthday present' for the baby.
- Make sure your firstborn overhears you saying lovely things about them to the baby e.g. 'you are so lucky to have ... as your brother/sister'.
- If you plan to increase their day care days, do this before the baby comes so it doesn't feel like such a big and sudden change on top of all of the adjustments they are experiencing at home.

Your Friends and Family

Even when surrounded by loved ones, you may feel lonely if none of them truly understand the enormity of the transition you are going through. Despite their best intentions, those without children usually don't 'get it', and those *with* children are often so busy with the demands of parenthood that they forget how tender and vulnerable the days, weeks and months following birth can be.

Assumptions, expectations and deeply entrenched dynamics all come into play when a baby is born. As doulas, we often see those closest to the birthing person being their biggest triggers, which can be due to the shift in your own personal identity as you become a mother. Your own parenting choices and the need to preserve and protect your energy may not be respected by those who feel entitled to dish out unsolicited advice or drop in for newborn cuddles whenever they fancy.

The good news is, unsolicited advice is rarely about you. It is often a way people validate their own parenting choices and decisions. If you do things the way *they* did, it means their way was right. This is where leaning into your intuition is helpful. Do what feels right for YOU. What works for others may not work for you, and that is okay, because no two mothers are the same, no two babies are the same, and no two mother–baby dyads are the same.

At the core of it all, people do want to help, they just need to be told how. This is where feeling confident to ask for help and learning how to put boundaries in place can be game changing to your postpartum experience.

A NOTE FOR FRIENDS AND FAMILY – HOW TO BE THE BEST VISITOR EVER

- Check if it's okay to stop by – impromptu visits aren't usually ideal in those early weeks.
- If you have even a hint of a sniffle, hold off on visiting until you are fully recovered.
- Always bring food – things that can go in the fridge/freezer and easily be reheated for dinner, as well as healthy snacks.
- Ask if you can pick up anything on your way – toilet paper, coffee, nappies etc.
- Wash your hands when you arrive.
- Delicious as newborns may be, avoid kissing them as their immune systems are incredibly vulnerable when they are so little. This is especially relevant if you have a cold sore, as the herpes virus is potentially fatal to newborns.
- Don't expect to hold the baby as they may need a nap or feed, or may be unsettled by the new noises and smells of excited visitors.
- Save the cigarettes or heavy perfume until after your visit.
- Make sure mum has eaten and has a warm drink or bottle of water by her side.
- Scan the house for any dirty cups or dishes and discreetly wash them. Tend to any other things that could be useful, such as taking out rubbish, folding laundry etc.
- Offer to water plants, walk dogs, take older children to the playground etc.
- Make it all about them. Even if you have had the worst day ever, leave that at the door and go in with open arms and ears, so you can support them in whatever capacity they need.
- Don't stay too long – unless you are getting into deep cleaning or deep conversation, an hour is usually enough.

Gentle Boundary Setting

In the first few weeks of having your baby at home, it's important to spend as much time as possible resting, feeding and bonding with your baby, to promote recovery and find your rhythm as a new family.

Some people spend their first few weeks post-birth in complete isolation, while others enjoy and look forward to the company of loved ones. Even the most well-intentioned visits can be stressful if they are prolonged, or coincide with feeding or napping schedules. Something to consider is whether you will feel comfortable breastfeeding in front of visitors and if not, how to manage that. Establishing breastfeeding and your confidence with it is more important than a visit from a partner's friend or distant relative in those early days.

This is where a food roster or meal train can be invaluable. It helps to mitigate the endless stream of visitors and invites them to show up with nourishing food. This is a great way of communicating your needs and you can include requests such as walking your dog, folding the laundry or picking up groceries. If asking for help still makes you feel uncomfortable (we get it, it takes time), ask a friend or doula to set up the meal train for you.

Boundary setting is simply a way of communicating your needs in a clear and practical manner. Those who don't respect or respond well to boundaries are often those who don't have clear boundaries themselves. This can be uncomfortable, however it is important to remain clear with your boundaries so you can preserve your precious energy as you recover from birth.

You may like to use the 'sandwich technique' when tackling difficult conversations, thus making it more digestible for the person on the receiving end.

E.g. 'I really love when you visit, however I need you to call first to check if it is a convenient time in case we are napping. We can't wait to see you.'

You may also wish to consider the following technique shared by Jenée Desmond-Harris.

How To Prioritise Your Precious Time and Energy:

1. Things you *need* to do   2. Things you *want* to do   3. Things *other people* want you to do.

You may find you don't often get to #3. This is okay. This is what it feels like to have boundaries.

Your Circle of Support

You may wish to consider using the following diagram to help you set up your postpartum circle of support, including who can visit and who can wait.

The specifics of your circle can vary, for example you may have a neighbour or acquaintance who you aren't particularly close with (yet) but who shows up for you with a meal, offers to hang out your laundry or walk your dog, as a surprising addition to your circle of support.

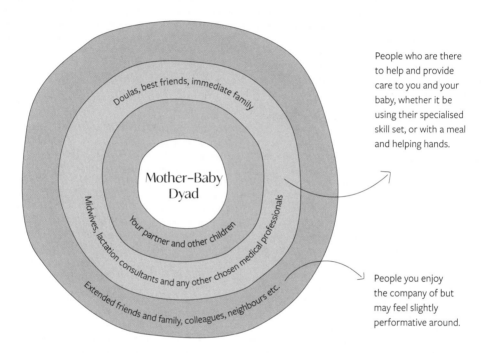

People who are there to help and provide care to you and your baby, whether it be using their specialised skill set, or with a meal and helping hands.

Doulas, best friends, immediate family

Mother–Baby Dyad

Your partner and other children

Midwives, lactation consultants and any other chosen medical professionals

Extended friends and family, colleagues, neighbours etc.

People you enjoy the company of but may feel slightly performative around.

LOVE LANGUAGES™

1

What makes you feel loved? Is it spending quality time with your partner, or is it receiving a back rub after a long day? Do kind and encouraging words fill your cup, or would you prefer someone helped you with the laundry? Or perhaps none of this matters if you aren't receiving gifts. It may be a combination of the above. These are your Love Languages™, a concept created by Gary Chapman in his book *The 5 Love Languages®: The Secret to Love That Lasts.*

Most people have one or two primary Love Languages™. When it comes to relationships, what many people don't understand is that our partners may not have the same Love Languages™ as us. It is important to learn the ways those closest to us wish to receive love. In doing so, we have a better understanding of their needs, which enables us to remain connected and show them that we do care, even through the haze of new parenthood.

Love Languages™ are relatable to both romantic and platonic relationships, as well as those we have with our families. They are useful for showing another that you love them, as well as reconnecting in times of conflict, or when you feel adrift.

Words of Affirmation

How it looks: Compliments, appreciation, validation, encouragement, loving text messages and handwritten notes.

Examples for the postpartum: 'You're such an amazing mother/ father', 'Thank you for folding the laundry', 'I know this is hard and you're doing a great job', 'I'm so proud of you'.

Obstacles: Criticism, forgetting to validate the enormous transition they've been through, being so consumed by your own exhaustion and endless 'to-do' list that you forget to communicate your love and appreciation.

2

Quality Time

How it looks: Uninterrupted one-on-one time, deep and meaningful conversation, being in one another's presence.

Examples for the postpartum: Sitting with your partner while they feed your baby, date nights, watching your favourite show together, going for a walk together, calling to check in throughout the day.

Obstacles: Work, baby and household chores getting in the way of connection, being on your phone while your partner is trying to talk to you, feeling like ships in the night as you tend to multiple children.

3

Receiving Gifts

How it looks: Thoughtful gifts on special occasions and 'just because'.

Examples for the postpartum: A 'push present', bringing home lunch or their favourite treat, ordering flowers or a 'self-care' gift online and having it delivered.

Obstacles: Thinking gifts need to be lavish to be appreciated, being so tired you forget to organise a big or little gift, focusing on gifts for baby and not for partners.

4

Acts of Service

How it looks: Helping with baby care and housework, doing things for your partner that you know they will appreciate.

Examples for the postpartum: Folding the laundry, taking care of nappy changes, cooking dinner, taking the baby or older kids so parent/s can rest, running a bath for the nursing parent.

Obstacles: Ignoring or forgetting requests for help, being too tired, not asking how you can help, allowing one parent to take on more responsibilities than the other.

5

Physical Touch

How it looks: Hugs, massage, hand holding, gentle, non-sexual touch, sexual intimacy.

Examples for the postpartum: Cuddling on the couch once your baby is asleep, offering them a foot or back-rub, giving affection enthusiastically, kissing your partner on the head as you walk past them feeding on the couch, lightly touching their arm while talking.

Obstacles: Feeling touched out, physical healing after birth, physical demands of parenthood, low libido.

YOUR NEST

Create a Sanctuary

Becoming a parent brings a lot of changes to your external world – sleep deprivation, caring for a new baby, navigating new roles and relationships, and so on. With the addition of the physical healing your body is going through and big emotions you may be feeling, retreating to a space that feels safe, promotes calm, sparks joy, and protects the precious mother–baby dyad, is going to benefit you and your family immensely. For this reason, we recommend turning your bedroom into a sanctuary. Here are some ideas from our years of experience as a mother and as postpartum doulas:

- Invest in the best quality mattress you can afford (we recommend a king or super king if you are planning to bed share), and ensure you have breathable cotton or linen sheets with extra pillows for support while you breastfeed.
- Make space next to your bed for a water bottle, snacks and nipple balm etc. Having a dedicated space (see our tip about a basket or caddy on page 45) for all your essentials will make them easier to find through the haze of night feeds and reduce the stress that can come from being surrounded by clutter.
- Adorning your walls with art or inspiring photos, diffusing essential oils, playing soothing music or bringing nature into your space with plants or flowers are other examples of how to set up your sanctuary.
- If you're someone who needs your space to be clean and de-cluttered in order to feel calm, be sure to include this in the conversations you have with your partner or support people, as this is something they can easily help with that will be game-changing for your state of mind and wellbeing. This applies to any other area of the home where you may wish to feed, rest and retreat.

Material Things to Support Your Recovery

Aside from a well-stocked pantry and a full freezer (covered in the following pages), there are a number of things we suggest to aid your physical recovery.

- Adult nappies (for the first week) and maternity pads or period undies (for the weeks following)
- Body oil (natural, plant based)
- Breast pads
- Cabbage leaves or hot/cold packs for breasts
- Compression shorts or belly binding
- Drink bottle with straw
- Hand-held night light or torch (so you can see in the dark when it's time for night feeds and nappy changes)
- Heat pack or hot water bottle
- Herbal pelvic steam (see page 125)

- Herbal Peri Pads (see page 122)
- Herbal sitz (see page 123)
- Herbal tea
- Insulated reusable cup or thermos
- Nipple balm
- Nursing bra or crop top
- One-handed snacks – see recipes on page 231
- Peri bottle
- Pillows (lots of them)
- PJs or a robe that makes you feel good
- Silicone breastmilk saver
- Warm and comfy socks and slippers

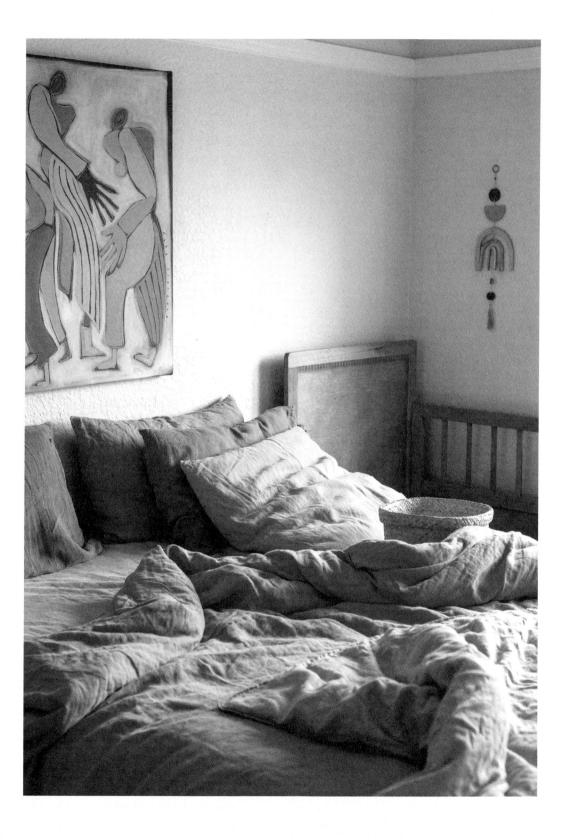

Your Postpartum Kitchen

When a mother is well nourished, so is her baby. This sentiment might seem *DUH* obvious, but do you know how often we walk into the homes of mothers we support and find plates of half-eaten, cold toast lying around? It's not easy to prioritise yourself after a night of little-to-no sleep, but we are here to remind you that you cannot pour from an empty cup. Mamas need and deserve to put their nutritional needs first and eat well during the postpartum, because the wellbeing and nourishment of a mother transfers to all of those around her.

As our cultural paradigm shifts and we bring reverence to the role that mothers play in the community, food can bring immense comfort and connection when cooked and shared between family, friends, neighbours and those we have only just met. Food brings us together like nothing else, and during your postpartum, honouring your beautiful, life-giving body and all that it has created is a great thing you can do for yourself. It's what you deserve. Food acts not just as fuel, but as medicine and nourishment on a soul-deep level.

Eating well will sustain and support your body, especially as it is adjusting, shifting and changing through the postpartum period, and it need not be complicated. It does require some planning, but once you create some simple routines with your eating habits, it will require less thought. In fact, that's why we were so excited to write this book: to offer you tangible guidance and practical support for all facets of motherhood, including self-nourishment.

On the next page you'll find a list of the most nutrient-dense foods to stock your pantry with before your baby arrives. These contain a multitude of food-based vitamins and minerals, and having them on hand will make food preparation much easier in the early months of motherhood. Studies have shown that when a breastfeeding mother's diet is rich in nutritious foods, it will transfer via breastmilk to her baby, which supports optimal physical and mental growth and development of the newborn.

Vaughne shares the following tips with the mamas she supports as a naturopath to make eating in the fourth trimester feel more manageable (and nourishing!). You'll also find a list of specific nutrients in the Nutrition and Herbal Support chapter (p. 109), which offers food sources for you to focus on based on your individual needs through your postpartum and beyond.

FILL YOUR FREEZER

During maternity leave, while nesting into your final weeks of pregnancy, is a great time to fill your freezer with warming and nourishing meals. Doing this will seriously lighten your load once baby arrives! It's also a great idea to ask friends and family, who want to support you, to make meals you can freeze, or start a meal train that can be delivered throughout the week. Meals and snacks that freeze well include soups, stews, broths, curries, slow-cooked meals using meat, legumes and root vegetables, rissoles and burger patties, pasta sauces, muffins, slices and bliss balls.

CHOOSE WARMING, EASILY DIGESTIBLE FOODS

Your digestive system is more sensitive in the weeks following birth and your body is recovering from the marathon effort of growing and birthing a whole other human. Many cultures believe that after labour, a woman's body is left feeling 'cold' and in need of warming meals to support recovery. Similarly, from a naturopathic perspective, foods cooked with warming herbs and spices yield therapeutic benefits that support breastmilk production, digestive function and the absorption and uptake of essential nutrients.

PROTEIN

Protein is an essential macronutrient required to support repair and recovery of muscles and cells, as well as regulate blood sugar and help us feel fuller for longer. Recent studies show that in the first six months of the postpartum period, exclusively breastfeeding mothers may require between 1.7–1.9 grams of protein per kilo of body weight, each day, to support their and their baby's nutritional needs. This might sound like a lot, but protein is abundant in so many delicious foods, such as legumes and beans, nuts, seeds and nut butters, tempeh, tofu, dairy, poultry, meat and fish. Aim to eat a palm-sized piece during each main meal and keep some protein-heavy snacks in your bag, next to your feeding chair and on your bedside table to keep you going throughout the day and night.

FATS

Fat is incredibly important to consume during pregnancy to fuel your baby's growing brain and neurological development, but did you know that it's just as important to boost fat consumption through your postpartum? Breastmilk is made up of over 50 per cent fat and human brains are composed of approximately 60 per cent fat, which makes it an essential macronutrient that we must consume in order to think and function at our healthiest. The important thing to focus on is the quality and variety of fats you're eating. Studies have shown that healthy fats, including those that are rich in omega-3, may reduce inflammation, lower the risk of blood clotting, support hormonal health and increase absorption of other nutrients. Trans fats and industrial vegetable oils are often processed and found in fried, baked and packaged junk foods, which studies have shown can increase inflammation in the body and the risk of postpartum depression. The best fats to eat liberally are found in nuts, seeds, avocado, olives, oily fish, eggs and extra-virgin olive oil.

CARBOHYDRATES

Carbohydrates are another essential macronutrient that fuel your brain and muscles, which is important for sleep-deprived and busy mothers, who also require the glucose found in carbs to produce the lactose that is found in breastmilk. Simple carbohydrates (or sugars) are often refined and do not contain adequate amounts of nutrients, starch or fibre, and so produce a greater spike in blood glucose and offer the body a shorter lasting source of energy. It's best to limit these foods, including white bread, cakes, lollies, pastries and soft drinks. Complex carbs on the other hand, provide a more sustained release of energy. The healthiest complex carbohydrates are unrefined plant foods that are high in fibre, such as brown rice, starchy vegetables, beans, legumes, and whole grains. To balance your blood sugar through the day, combine carbs with a source of protein and fat, such as sourdough toast loaded with avocado and goat's feta.

FIBRE

After your baby has spent the better half of nine months squashing your organs, your digestive system may need some time to recover and get back into a healthy groove. Ensuring that you are eating enough fibre will help regulate your bowel function by bulking the stool and making it easier to pass. Fibre-rich foods such as vegetables, fruit, whole grains, nuts, seeds and legumes can also support blood sugar regulation, as it helps to slow digestion which can curb sugar cravings and stabilise your energy. Our gut microbiome also benefits from fibre, as some contain prebiotics which feed the healthy bacteria in our intestines which are important for optimal digestive health.

Postpartum Pantry List

GRAINS & FLOURS

Whole grains are the best form to choose, as they contain the most nutrients and are the least refined. Many of these are gluten free.

- Amaranth (grains, puffed)
- Buckwheat (grains, flour)
- Cassava flour
- Coconut flour
- Green banana flour
- Oats (steel-cut, flour – rolled oats can be quicker for cooking)
- Quinoa (grains, flakes, puffed)
- Rice – white and brown (grains, flakes, puffed)
- Rye
- Spelt
- Wild rice

NUTS & SEEDS

Nuts are a wonderful source of protein and healthy fats to keep you satiated and help to stabilise your blood sugar and energy through the day. Enjoy raw or dry roasted, as well as in 'butter' form without added sugar or refined vegetable oils.

- Almonds
- Brazil nuts
- Cashew nuts
- Chia seeds
- Coconut (flaked or shredded)
- Hemp seeds
- Linseeds (flax seeds)
- Macadamia nuts
- Pepitas (pumpkin seeds)
- Pistachio nuts
- Sesame seeds
- Sunflower seeds
- Walnuts

BEANS & LEGUMES

Beans are best soaked in water overnight with 1 teaspoon of bicarbonate of soda (baking soda) to help break down anti-nutrients such as phytates, making them less likely to cause digestive disturbances.

- Black beans
- Black beluga lentils
- Butter beans
- Cannellini beans
- Chickpeas
- French green/puy lentils
- Mung beans (split are easier to cook)
- Red lentils

MEAT, EGGS AND DAIRY

Opt for organic, grass-fed, pasture raised or wild caught where financially possible, as these animals are not fed synthetic hormones and antibiotics. These are commonly fed to animals living on conventional farms and their living standards are often much lower than sustainable farms.

- Butter
- Chicken and beef broth, or bones to make it
- Eggs
- Fish – sardines, mackerel, anchovies, salmon, trout
- Goat's cheese
- Liver
- Meats – beef, lamb, kangaroo, chicken, turkey
- Parmesan

FERMENTED FOODS

These are a great source of probiotics, which support the growth of healthy gut bacteria, improved digestion and breakdown of nutrients from your food and supplements.

- Kefir
- Kimchi
- Kombucha
- Miso
- Pickled vegetables
- Sauerkraut
- Yoghurt (choose a natural, sugar-free option)

OILS & BUTTERS

Unrefined, cold-pressed oils are best. Avoid refined vegetable oils which are inflammatory to the body, and opt for grass-fed dairy products.

- Avocado oil
- Butter (if you can tolerate dairy)
- Cacao butter
- Coconut oil
- Extra-virgin olive oil
- Ghee (clarified butter)
- Hemp oil
- Linseed oil
- Walnut oil

HERBS & SPICES

Many herbs and spices contain therapeutic properties to support digestion, lactation, blood sugar regulation, reduce inflammation and provide warmth during the postpartum period.

- Aniseed
- Black pepper
- Cardamom
- Cayenne
- Cinnamon
- Clove
- Coriander
- Cumin
- Fennel
- Fenugreek
- Ginger
- Nutmeg
- Orange peel
- Turmeric

DRIED FRUIT

Choose sulphur free – this additive has been known to cause reactivity in some people, such as asthma, headaches, skin rashes, digestive upset and nausea. Avoid ingredients 220, 221, 222, 223, 224, 225.

- Apricots
- Chinese 'jujube' dates
- Figs
- Goji berries
- Medjool dates (these can also be found fresh in your local grocer's fridge)
- Pears
- Peaches
- Prunes

PLANT MILKS

Try to avoid plant milks that contain refined vegetable oils, gums, thickeners and sugar, as these can be inflammatory to the body.

- Almond
- Coconut
- Hemp
- Macadamia
- Oat

SWEETENERS

These sugar alternatives offer a lower glycaemic load to better support blood sugar stability, while providing other nutrients that refined and conventional sugars do not. A little goes a long way, so use sparingly in your cooking to add a pop of sweetness.

- Blackstrap molasses (plant based iron source)
- Coconut sugar (better alternative to conventional sugar as contains prebiotic inulin)
- Local honey (raw, unpasteurised)
- 100% pure maple syrup (avoid maple 'flavoured' syrups which are high in sugar)
- Stevia (choose raw, organic in green form to avoid artificial additives)

OTHER ITEMS FROM THE HEALTH FOOD STORE:

- **Nutritional yeast** – a plant based source of vitamin B12 which can be sprinkled on meals as a cheese alternative, or added to soups and stews for flavour.
- **Sea vegetables** (wakame, kelp flakes, dulse, nori sheets etc.) – a plant based source of iodine to support thyroid health. Can be enjoyed sprinkled on food or wrapped around pickled vegetables and avocado as a snack.
- **Psyllium husk and slippery elm** – a source of bulking fibre to help with postpartum constipation. Can be taken in capsule form or powder added to water or smoothies.
- **Raw cacao & cacao nibs** – a superfood source of magnesium and antioxidants which can be added to smoothies, healthy baked or raw treats for a chocolate fix.
- **Grass-fed collagen & gelatine powder** – a source of protein and amino acids which is essential for maintaining the normal structure, strength and integrity of connective tissue such as skin, bones, cartilage and blood vessels. These can be added to smoothies, oats, healthy baked or raw treats and gummies (gelatine is a thickener so makes the perfect addition to healthy jelly and panna cotta for extra gut-loving goodness).
- **Bone broth** (fresh, powder or concentrate) – rich in collagen, gelatine, amino acids and minerals which support postpartum healing. Enjoy as is or add to soups, stews, casseroles, curries, sauces and gravy for added nutritional value.

Hot Tip for Food Storage:

Store your pantry staples, leftovers and water in glass and stainless steel jars and containers. Avoid storing food in plastic and always transfer to a glass or ceramic dish before heating, as warming plastic can cause it to leach chemicals – notably endocrine disruptors – into your food which is detrimental to your health. This can include heating leftover soup in a plastic container in the microwave or using a plastic spatula to mix and flip food in a hot frypan. The same goes for Teflon coating. The jury is out as to just how dangerous it is, but we say it's best to avoid where possible. Learn more about the chemical load caused by conventional cleaning and beauty products on page 43.

Hot Tip for Food Shopping:

When it comes to choosing foods that are better for your health or for the environment, but also fit into your weekly budget, there are many resources out there to help you navigate this.

Each year, the US Environmental Working Group (EWG) releases a list of foods called the 'Clean 15' and 'Dirty Dozen', which provides a general guideline for foods with a lower toxic load (non-organic), and others that are recommended to eat organically. In Australia, we have different farming practices and pesticide use, but we can use the list as a rough guide.

Where possible, buy produce from small, organic farmers and markets to support your health and the local economy. Sometimes this can be cheaper (and tastier) than buying from supermarkets!

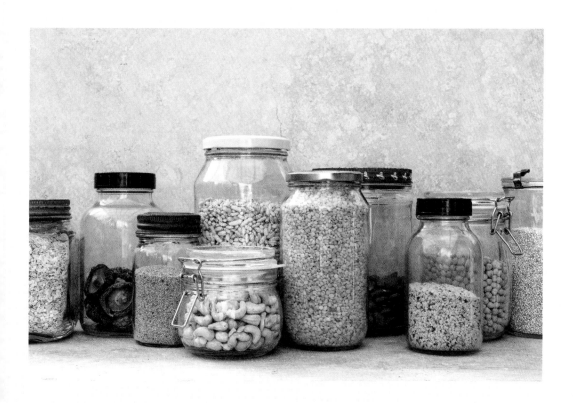

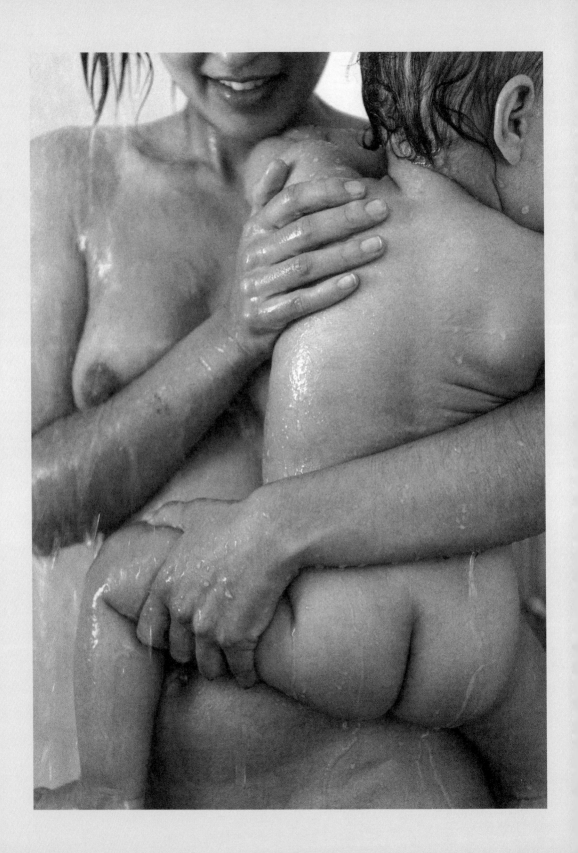

Chemicals in the Home

The skin is our body's largest organ and absorbs what we apply topically, such as moisturiser and sunscreen, as well as things like dry shampoo and perfume. Likewise, our entire respiratory system is highly sensitive to chemicals and toxins in our environment. Just as we inhale second-hand smoke and pollution, we inhale chemicals that we spray over ourselves and our homes, including air fresheners, shower cleaner and bug spray.

Over eighty thousand man-made chemicals have never been tested for their impact on human health, and many of them are in conventional home and beauty products, which we are unknowingly exposing ourselves and our children to each and every day.

An increasing number of studies show how detrimental these chemicals are to our health, and how continuous exposure can wreak havoc on our hormones, fertility, nervous system and immune health.

Synthetic chemicals including fragrances and preservatives are found in everything from hand and body wash, hair products, moisturisers and sunscreens, make-up and baby-care products, to laundry and washing detergents, bathroom cleaners, surface and room sprays, candles and more. Using a multitude of these products can place an enormous burden on your body's natural detoxification systems, causing them to accumulate and lead to a number of health concerns.

'Endocrine disrupting chemicals' (EDCs) mimic and interfere with the way hormones work. They act on your endocrine system – a series of glands that produce and secrete natural hormones – and can affect fertility for both you and your unborn child, in both males and females. It can also lead to health concerns such as asthma, eczema and other skin irritation and allergies. They have even been shown to increase the risk of cancer.

Despite studies now showing a vast number of these chemicals to be unsafe, they continue to be used in abundance in the beauty world. Some of the most common toxins include:

Formaldehyde: Traditionally used in the embalming of dead bodies, it is also used in hair straightening treatments, soap and nail polish. The greatest risk of toxicity is through inhalation, which can cause skin redness and itching plus irritation of the eyes, nose, and throat, as well as cancer risk.

Phthalates: Found in more than 70 per cent of deodorants, perfumes, hair and skincare products, phthalates (pronounced thalates) have been linked to serious hormonal issues, altered genital development, low sperm count, infertility, some cancers and more.

Other major chemicals to avoid: Commercial cleaning and hygiene products that include chemicals such as bleach, ammonia, sodium hydroxide, chlorine, synthetic fragrances, aluminium, parabens, sulphates, mineral oils, nanoparticles, Polyethylene Glycol (PEG), petroleum.

Some of these chemicals are also used in the production of clothing, fabrics and furniture. For example, formaldehyde and phthalates are applied to fabrics to enhance softening, wrinkle and shrink resistance.

From a health perspective, chemicals, particularly dyes, can cause allergic skin reactions or contact dermatitis, which is why it is recommended to wash all new clothing and fabrics before they are worn in order to get rid of any residual chemicals. Better yet, shopping for vintage or second-hand clothing and sharing 'hand-me-down' baby and children's clothes is a great way to support the environment when fast fashion is placing such a strain on our planet. Where possible, opt for organic materials such as linen, sustainably farmed cotton and hemp coloured with natural dye to reduce the chemical load for your family.

Two resources we recommend when researching your skincare and household products include *The Chemical Maze* (book and app), alongside the Environmental Working Group website.

YOUR BABY

With the recent and increasing commodification of motherhood, there are lots of mixed messages about what you really need for your baby. What you will realise when you bring them home, is that all your baby really needs is you.

Heidi Sze says in her book *Nurturing Your New Life*, 'There are nifty creations that can make your life easier, but nothing can tame the primal need for contact and milk. Some infants require advanced medical care to thrive, and we are fortunate to live in a time when this is available. But generally speaking, the empowering and overwhelming truth is that babies only need you. They need you all day and sometimes all night, no matter how tired you are, and with no regard for your modern-world obligations.'

We have created a list of things that – in our experience as a mother and as doulas – we deem essential and potentially helpful for your babe in those first few weeks and months at home.

DEFINITE DOZEN:

- Attend a baby First Aid and CPR course
- Baby wipes
- Burp cloth
- Car seat
- Cot and/or bassinet and/or co-sleeper
- First aid kit
- Nappies
- Nappy rash cream (natural)
- Onesies (with fold-down mittens)
- Pram and/or baby carrier
- Singlets
- Swaddles.

THINGS YOU MIGHT FIND USEFUL:

- Baby bath
- Baby bath care products (natural)
- Baby monitor
- Baby sleep sack
- Baby towel
- Beanie
- Breast/chestfeeding chair
- Breast pump
- Bottles, steriliser and brush
- Bouncer-net
- Cardigan and/or jumper
- Fitted sheets (for baby bed)
- Formula
- Humidifier
- Infant lounger
- Leggings
- Nail clippers
- Nappy bin
- Pacifier
- Play mat
- Socks
- Thermometer
- White noise machine.

Hot Tip #1: Create a basket that you can move around the house with you, so you have everything you need at hand. Fill it with nappies, wipes, burp cloth, towel or change mat, swaddle, nipple balm, two changes of clothes for baby, drink bottle and snacks.

Hot Tip #2: You don't *need* a change table. If you have space, you can set up a changing mat on a chest of drawers, dining table, couch or living room floor. Bring your basket of goodies and you're good to go!

Hot Tip #3: You don't *need* a nappy bag. Find yourself a comfortable backpack that has a side pocket for your drink bottle, or use any bag you already have at home, such as a sturdy tote bag with internal pockets. In it, put a drawstring bag filled with nappies, wipes, a towel to change baby on and two sets of baby clothes. Keep the burp cloth, nipple balm, swaddle, baby toys and your snacks in the backpack/tote bag too.

Hot Tip #4: The Stokke Tripp Trapp® highchair is revered not only for its style, but also its practicality as it is adjustable for all ages, and supports children's feet when they eat. There is a newborn attachment that clips on so you can engage with baby while you are cooking or eating.

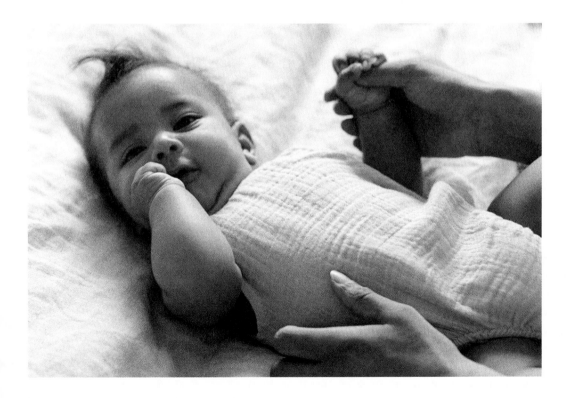

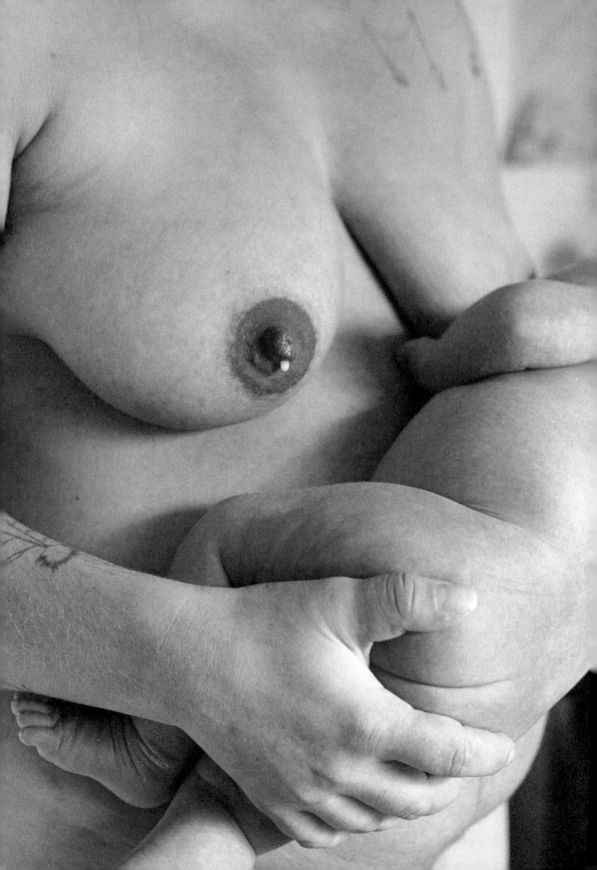

A BRIEF
GUIDE TO

CHAPTER TWO

BREAST-
FEEDING

As we acknowledge our scope of practice, we have consulted, collaborated and had our information fact-checked by Amy Sherer – a registered midwife and International Board Certified Lactation Consultant (IBCLC), with almost twenty years of experience in the maternity sector. She believes there are fundamental issues with the maternity system in Australia, especially in reference to evidence-based and accurate information. She has provided us with a deeper level of knowledge based on the most up-to-date research, and she uses clever anecdotes to help us better understand the complex world of breastfeeding and lactation.

Our breast tissue is an enormously clever and complex system containing glandular tissue, alveoli, milk ducts, nerve endings, ligaments, fat, blood and lymph. Contrary to common myth, milk production is not dependent on breast size.

Our bodies are incredibly intuitive and respond to breast and nipple stimulation by sending a signal to the pituitary gland to release prolactin (the milk making hormone) and oxytocin (the milk ejection hormone). This in turn signals your breasts to make more milk and eject it into your baby's mouth. How incredibly clever!

That being said, the first few weeks of learning to breastfeed can be harder than birth itself. If you are able to persevere, once you turn a corner you may find it to be a magical and rewarding bonding experience that has innumerable benefits for both you and your baby.

As doulas, we often see new mums come home from the hospital bewildered and confused about breastfeeding. The common experience is that women have received conflicting advice by different midwives and other care providers in the hospital, and often head home feeling unsure about what to do and who to listen to.

This, according to Amy Sherer, is because 'current research can take years to filter down to institutional level where it is passed on to parents, hence the common experience of conflicting advice in maternity care.'

Another thing we notice consistently with new mums is their surprise at how frequently newborns want to feed. This one doesn't discriminate. No matter how your baby was born or what level of support you have, newborns are demanding and most of them don't adhere to the schedules of the modern parent.

We aren't saying any of this to scare you, but rather to encourage you to arm yourself with information and support so that you have the knowledge and confidence you need to embark on a successful breastfeeding journey.

We highly recommend reading a breastfeeding book in the final month of your pregnancy that also educates you around biologically normal infant behaviour so you know what to expect with your baby's behaviour patterns, crying, fussing and feeding. This will help you navigate the onslaught of well-intentioned advice, giving you the power to listen to what feels right (hello intuition!) and ignore what doesn't. There are numerous resources available – we will list our favourites in the Resources section (page 232).

When we asked our wider community for their advice for new parents, the second most popular response (after investing in your postpartum) was that you book a lactation consultant in the first week of being home. Amy advises to look for a *currently registered* IBCLC. They are available both publicly and privately, with most countries having local breastfeeding associations and/or free hotlines you can call. Lactation consultants have the skill and knowledge to look at each mother–baby dyad holistically and individually. They are often also qualified midwives with many years of maternity experience under their belts.

What we share in the pages that follow doesn't by any means replace a good breastfeeding book or lactation consultant, but will hopefully serve as a guide and morale booster, to see you through as you learn how to breastfeed your tiny human.

The three biggest factors that influence breastfeeding failure or success are:

1. Support and rest
2. Quality of education and accurate information
3. Cultural norms regarding breastfeeding.

The three main factors that influence ongoing milk production are:

1. Milk removal (breastfeeding and/or expressing) and nipple stimulation (in the way of suckling, grabbing, head bobbing, nuzzling etc.)
2. Hormones (these vary uniquely from person to person)
3. Adequate rest, hydration, nutrition and support.

A TYPICAL BREASTFEEDING TIMELINE

PREGNANCY:

Breast tissue grows only two times in your life: puberty and pregnancy, the latter being when the most significant changes occur. You will notice not only a change in breast size, but also in the colour and shape of your areola and nipples (they get darker which helps baby to find them) and your veins may become more prominent. It's important to note the degree of changes have minimal to no bearing on the outcome of your milk production.

Colostrum production begins from around 16 weeks of pregnancy. Colostrum is a low-volume nutrient-dense substance that may appear thick like honey or be watery and even different colours from one person to the next. Colostrum is tailored to your baby's specific needs and contains the immune blueprint for your baby's lifetime.

You may wish to discuss the advantages of antenatal hand expressing with your healthcare provider. Antenatal expression can be especially beneficial for those who develop gestational diabetes or who have pre-existing diabetes. A good place to start with general information on this topic is via the Australian Breastfeeding Association. We recommend their article 'Antenatal Expression of Colostrum'. When seeking advice on this topic it is important to ensure your health practitioner is up to date with the latest advice and research and is also qualified to advise you on whether it is safe for you to hand express under your specific circumstances.

BIRTH TO 8 HOURS AFTER BIRTH:

In ideal circumstances, baby should be placed skin-to-skin on your chest immediately after birth. If this is not possible – such as after neonatal or obstetric emergencies – aim to initiate skin-to-skin contact as soon as you are able. Ask your care provider to assist you if this is not something you feel confident with.

Babies are often very alert in the first hour following birth; this is the prime circumstance for a baby to perform the breast crawl before nursing for the first time.

The Breast Crawl:

Immediately after birth, your baby should be placed naked on your bare chest. The first hour post-birth is known as the 'golden hour' – when oxytocin is at an all-time high. Skin-to-skin action further supports the production of oxytocin which plays an important role in driving prolactin, the hormone that produces breastmilk. Given the right circumstances, your baby should perform the breast crawl. This is when the baby finds your breasts all on their own (which to them, smell like the amniotic fluid they have been suspended in until now). They will push with their feet to do this, which in turn helps your uterus to contract and expel the placenta. The human body really is a miracle.

8 TO 24 HOURS AFTER BIRTH:

Your baby may be very sleepy during this period. It is not necessary to wake them for a feed unless it has been more than 6 hours, or it is medically indicated to do so (such as with premature, very small babies, or those requiring blood sugar monitoring).

Feeding Cues and Reflexes:

- **Rooting reflex** – when baby turns their head towards you or tries to suckle onto anything that brushes their cheek (in hope that it's a nipple).
- **Sucking on hands** – 'Maybe that's where the milk comes from?!'
- **Lip smacking and tongue sucking** – this one is contentious as it is not always a sign of hunger (but it can be). You know your baby best and will soon figure out if they are smacking their lips because they are hungry or because they enjoy the sensation.
- **Poking the tongue out** – baby may simply be practising this for fun, or it may be a feeding cue.

24 TO 48 HOURS AFTER BIRTH:

From around 24 hours it is important to feed your baby more frequently.

Some feeds may occur in clusters or very close together, or they may be longer with lots of swapping or 'switch feeding' (swapping from one breast to the other). It is important to remember that some feeds will be to satiate hunger while others will be for comfort and security as the baby seeks to regulate their nervous system following their own transition from foetus to baby. Babies have no concept that they are separate from you at this early stage and require loads of reassurance. Allowing your baby to suckle as often as they need to will comfort them and stimulate your breasts to produce milk. Suckling also provides babies with exercises that support brain development and oral development.

2 TO 3 DAYS AFTER BIRTH:

Your baby may feed in longer, more regular blocks of time, or have long stretches of fussing and/or feeding constantly or around the clock as they bring in your milk. Your colostrum may become more watery as it increases in volume, water, lactose (milk sugar) and fat. This is sometimes called 'transitional milk'.

Everything you've read will have told you that breastfeeding isn't painful and it shouldn't hurt, but your nipples may feel sensitive from all the sudden action they are experiencing. This will pass, but if you notice any cracks, blisters, bleeding or bruises, it's important to ensure baby's latch is correct, to mitigate further damage and other associated problems. If your nipples are becoming damaged it is likely because baby is not latching well. This may mean they aren't receiving enough milk, which will also affect your supply. There is only so much that can be communicated through a book or the internet, so if your intuition tells you that your latch isn't correct, see a lactation consultant immediately. One breastfeeding problem can lead to a cascade of issues, so it is important to seek help and nip any small issues in the bud.

Weight Gains and Losses:

It is normal for babies to lose up to 10 per cent (and sometimes a little more) of their birth weight in the days before your milk comes in. The aim is for babies to regain their birth weight by approximately days 10 to 14, and to put on around 20 to 30 grams per day thereafter. Some babies get off to a slower start and others deviate from the recommended weight gains for many reasons. Information about normal weight gain with an insight to percentile charts can be found via the Australian Breastfeeding Association website.

To Time Feeds or Not To Time Feeds?

For some, timing feeds can be detrimental to your mental health and make you worry if your baby's feeding pattern changes. While there may be instances where you need to time feeds – such as if your baby has jaundice or is generally not showing an interest in feeding – you should feed as frequently and for as long as your baby needs and offer both breasts during a feed cycle (unless they don't want it or a lactation consultant has advised you otherwise). This is known as 'feeding on demand'. Remember, babies don't know the hands on a clock, as they function only by instinct in their first few weeks of life.

'As adults, we grab a cup of tea, a glass of water, a sweet, a snack. We respond to our personal cues and we're flexible depending on time of day, the temperature, our mood, our energy levels. Many go to bed with a glass of water or sip from a bottle throughout the day. I don't know any adults that look at their watch and say, "Only 30 minutes till my next sip of water or mint! Not long now." But yet we expect teeny growing babies to be governed by this artificial notion of time.'

– Emma Pickett, The Dangerous Game of the Feeding Interval Obsession

3 TO 5 DAYS AFTER BIRTH:

Your baby may continue to want to nurse around the clock. This is around the time where they become more motivated by hunger rather than just the need to suckle. This is often coined 'cluster feeding' and if you aren't expecting it, it may cause you to question your supply. Hang in there, and know that your baby is doing exactly what they are supposed to.

Once your milk comes in, your breasts may feel rock hard or become engorged. If baby is having trouble latching due to engorgement, it is important to express a little before feeding, to make it easier for your baby to latch and to prevent nipple damage. Milk may remain yellow for another week or so if it still contains colostrum.

Once your milk is in, your baby may continue to enjoy frequent and lengthy feeds, especially in the first two to four weeks. This is biologically normal and is a continuation of the baby's adjustment to the world – they are feeding for comfort as well as nutrition. Your baby may often fall asleep at the breast due to the presence of melatonin in your milk and because sucking switches on the parasympathetic (rest and digest) nervous system. While once believed to be 'bad habit' forming, science is now showing that falling asleep at the breast is a biological norm, and another case of your baby doing exactly what they are supposed to do.

Counting Dirty Diapers:

Counting diapers is a useful way of ensuring your baby is getting what they need. You know what is going in by what is coming out. A general rule of thumb in the first five days is that the number of dirty nappies should correlate to how many days old your baby is e.g. Day 1 = 1 wee and 1 poo, Day 2 = 2 wees and 2 poos, and so on.

The first few poos will be black, tarry meconium. As milk composition changes, poop may become green and seedy like pesto, followed by numerous strangely pleasant, sweet-smelling, yellow, watery and seedy poos (a little bit like mustard or satay). From day five onward you may be changing up to 10 nappies every day, doing the math and counting how quickly you will go broke if your baby continues to poo so much. Rest assured, their poo will become less watery and then gradually reduce, which can be a good time to switch to cloth nappies if you plan to (but only if your mental health can handle the literal load).

When babies have formula milk the gut transit time is slower and digestion is different to breastmilk, therefore the baby may not poo as much.

5 DAYS TO 6 MONTHS AFTER BIRTH:

As your breasts relax you may wonder if your supply has reduced, but worry not, breast fullness is not a reliable measure of milk supply, nor is leakage! If your baby appears satisfied after a feed and has consistent wee and poo nappies, this is usually a sign that your supply is as it should be.

It's also important to note that the amount you pump is not a reliable indicator of milk supply. Babies are much more efficient at removing milk from breasts than machines are, as pumps don't stimulate the neuro-hormonal reactions in your breasts and brain that your baby does, therefore the amount you are able to pump isn't necessarily indicative of how much your baby is getting.

The number one most reliable sign of milk transfer is hearing regular, audible swallows at the breast; this is easier to hear once your supply increases and you may need a trained professional to help you identify it.

Given that you have the right support, adequate nutrition and rest, and drink plenty of water and herbal teas, your body will continue to be the sole source of food for your baby until they are around six months of age, as it contains all the nutrients and building blocks they need for optimal development. Pretty amazing huh? As they get older, they will continue to nurse not only due to hunger but also for comfort, pain relief through teething and sickness, connection and sleep. It is important to know that your milk remains nutritious beyond six months and adjusts composition alongside baby's needs for their age.

Breastmilk is a living substance and your body produces different milk at different times of the day. At night, your breastmilk contains more melatonin (the sleep hormone), and during the day it contains more cortisol (the waking hormone). You will notice that a boob in the mouth is the best solution to any major or minor incident, from vaccinations to falling over at the playground and everything in between.

6 MONTHS ONWARD:

Your baby will begin to explore solids alongside breastmilk, as you slowly increase the amount of food they eat and reduce the amount of milk they drink.

Your body will continue to make milk that is customised to your baby's needs, based on the miracle that is the 'backwash effect' (absorption of saliva by the areola) and our innate desire to cover our babies in kisses.

When it's time to introduce solids, check out the book *Milk to Meals* by Luka McCabe and Carley Mendes, and the *Solid Starts* app.

'When your baby breastfeeds, a vacuum is created and their saliva is sucked back into your nipple along with important information about their personal immune status. It travels "upstream" to the receptors in your mammary glands, which rapidly respond by producing specific antibodies to meet your baby's unique need. These antibodies are then delivered back to your baby via new made-to-order milk. It means that if you or your baby have picked up a virus or some pathogenic bacteria, their saliva will inform your memory gland receptors to create the specific antibodies required to help fight them. The antibodies then travel through your breastmilk to your baby. Not only that, but by kissing your baby, you pick up and consume viruses or pathogenic bacteria your baby has come in contact with. Your body then creates antibodies to fight those pathogens, which the baby receives directly through your breastmilk. Writing up and delivering the perfect prescription.'

CARLEY MENDES, OH BABY SCHOOL OF HOLISTIC NUTRITION

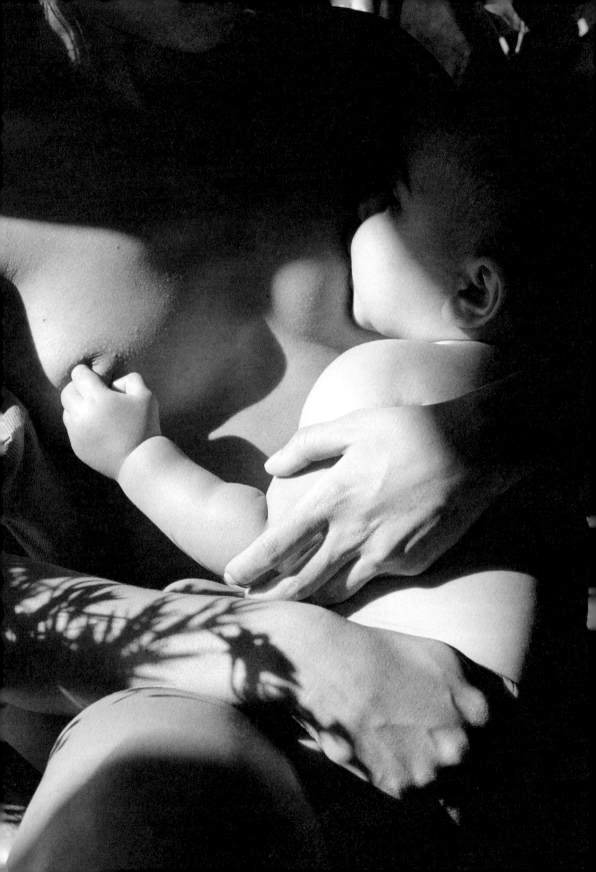

TIPS FOR COMMON BREASTFEEDING CHALLENGES

Under Supply

Typically, low supply stems from inadequate or infrequent milk removal, but can also be due to medical conditions such as a history of breast surgery or hormonal disease. Other factors that may contribute are lack of rest, relaxation, poor nutrition and low hydration (we know, we know, we say this a lot but these things really are important!). Research has shown that lack of support is also a major hindrance to breastfeeding sustainability and longevity.

Because insufficient breastmilk can be caused by a myriad of reasons, it is important to seek out a holistic assessment by a lactation consultant if you suspect you have an under-supply. Treatments such as topping up with formula, or pumping after a feed are often introduced without addressing the root cause of the problem. This increased separation between mother and baby changes the way baby feeds and behaves at the breast. The 'top-up trap' often leads to under supply and can deplete baby's feeding skills over time.

Over Supply

Over supply is characterised by baby gagging, coughing, gasping and frequently coming off the breast. This can cause babies to adjust their latch, causing nipple damage as they try to cope with the waterfall of milk. Some babies even make clicking sounds at the breast, which can be misdiagnosed as an oral tie or air swallowing. In extreme cases, over supply may cause breast refusal or babies may have symptoms of lactose overload (different to lactose intolerance).

Forceful milk ejection reflex (MER) is usually present in cases of over supply. This is where the hormonal pathways that eject milk into the baby's mouth get too excited. The stimulation of the baby at the breast triggers oxytocin (which causes contractions in the uterus and the breast) to squirt out milk. This can also occur when over supply isn't an issue.

Over supply and forceful MER can be challenging and upsetting especially if the baby appears to not be enjoying the feeding experience. This lactation challenge requires early intervention. In the meantime you may try and feed in a semi-reclined position that helps to slow the flow of milk (although this can be challenging for those with larger breasts). Ensuring your baby has a deep latch, and allowing them to have breaks from the breast as needed, is important to avoid a feeding strike.

Engorgement

Engorged breasts happen due to increased blood and lymphatic flow to your breasts in the days following birth. They can also happen at any stage during your breastfeeding journey, due to inadequate milk removal. It can feel like hell and prevent your baby from being able to latch properly, resulting in nipple damage which is a slippery slope into more serious breastfeeding problems. Sudden or ongoing engorgement is usually a sign of a deeper problem and may predispose you to mastitis and plugged ducts. Engorgement or milk stasis in the breast can also cause your supply to decrease as the body has a clever control mechanism to prevent you from filling up and up and up. Gently hand expressing or using a pump on a low setting before each feed will help to ease engorgement, making it easier for your baby to latch and therefore less painful for you.

You can hand express in the shower, however it's not always practical to shower before every feed, so we recommend using a bowl of warm-hot water and face washers, or a heat pack. Heat, in combination with expressing, will open up the blood vessels in the breast to help blood, lymph and milk flow. Post-feed, placing cold cabbage leaves, ice, or a cold compress in your bra provides enormous relief.

Nipple Damage

Nipple damage usually presents itself in the way of sore, cracked, bleeding or blistered nipples. It is usually caused by a poor latch (which can be due to engorged breasts, incorrect positioning or in rarer cases a tongue tie), but can also be caused by incorrect use of breast pumps, and occasionally medical issues such as dermatitis or thrush.

The easiest way to treat most forms of nipple damage is by correcting the latch. Sometimes we need help finding the right position for our babies and our breasts, which is why we recommend booking a lactation consultant for the first week at home with your baby. What works for others may not work for you, and what has worked for previous babies may not work for current or future ones.

A lactation consultant will approach nipple pain by assessing three main contributing factors (all of which may be exacerbating each other in various combinations).

1. Baby factors – latch, oral structures and variables that affect baby's feeding skills.
2. Mother factors – dermatological issues or incorrect use of a pump.
3. Your nervous system – your response to pain, trauma history and emotional states.

While there are a number of products that can provide short-term relief (such as Silverettes, nipple balms and hydrogel breast pads), they do not address the root cause of nipple damage.

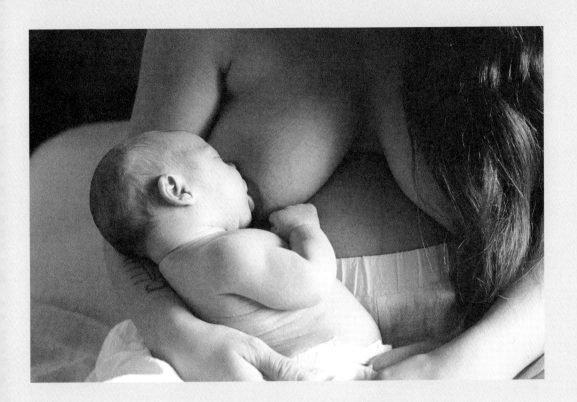

Vasospasm

Vasospasm is when the blood vessels in your nipple and breast constrict and can range from mild discomfort to extreme pain. Vasospasm is typically exacerbated by cold, nipple stimulation (e.g. in the shower) and breastfeeding.

Vasospasm is characterised by a deep burning or radiating throbbing pain into the breast and chest, and can be mistaken for nipple or breast thrush. In some instances the nipple may turn white or deep purple. Treatment involves addressing the root cause of the issue: attachment to the breast. Other treatments may involve avoiding cold sensation and encouraging warming of the nipples. There is strong evidence to suggest that magnesium supplementation, fish or algae oil capsules (containing essential fatty acids) or evening primrose oil (containing gamma linoleic acid) may improve blood vessel relaxation. In extreme cases a doctor may need to prescribe blood pressure medication to make feeding tolerable.

Inverted and Flat Nipples

It's not fair to judge a nipple by its appearance. Similar to tongue ties, merely the presence of a flat or inverted nipple does not indicate that the baby will not be able to latch successfully. However, people with flat or inverted nipples may require additional support to establish breastfeeding. This is where early intervention and sometimes the use of nipple shields may be beneficial.

A Note about Nipple Shields:

Nipple shields are a soft, silicone teat-shaped device that sits over the nipple and areola, originally designed to use on breasts with flat or inverted nipples, to create a protrusion for the baby to latch on to. They may be a long or short-term solution for a baby who is struggling to latch.

Shields can be an absolute game changer, but because they create a barrier between mother and baby, they may affect your milk supply which is why it is essential to seek guidance when using them.

Nipple shields are often used as a solution to nipple damage, however that is not their intended use.

Amy's advice if you choose shields to cope with nipple damage:

1. Ensure they are applied correctly. This is essential to ensure they don't slip and further damage the nipple. Most shields must be inverted and create a vacuum at the nipple base to ensure milk is easily transferred to baby. Check the manufacturer's guide to be sure.
2. Ensure baby is correctly latched over the shield, so as to not cause further damage and ensure milk is removed and transferred to the baby.
3. Book a review with an IBCLC to address the underlying issues, and to prevent further issues that may be caused by nipple shields.

Blocked Ducts and Mastitis

A plugged duct is an area of the breast where the flow of breastmilk is obstructed. It can feel like a tender lump or spot in the breast. These can result in a white spot or nipple blister where the milk is trying to exit the breast, sometimes referred to as a milk bleb. Plugged ducts can be an indication that you are at a higher risk for mastitis.

Mastitis is an obstruction and/or inflammation of the breast, which often involves symptoms similar to a plugged duct, but also includes a red area on the breast and is usually accompanied by a fever and body aches. When it first begins, it can feel like you've been struck by the flu. Blocked ducts, milk blisters and mastitis can be caused by a mixture of influences including immune health, inadequate milk removal (skipped feeds, poor latch), and infection by way of bacteria due to nipple damage. If left untreated mastitis may lead to a breast abscess and systemic illness.

Holistic ways to support yourself during an infection and to prevent future mastitis:

- Drink plenty of water throughout the day to keep yourself hydrated and your breastmilk flowing. Herbal teas such as lemon balm and chamomile will help relax your nervous system and promote let-down.
- Echinacea tincture to support your immune system and lymphatic drainage of the breast. Take 2 droppers/ 2 ml every two hours throughout the day during an acute phase, and continue to dose 2 ml, three times daily for two days after symptoms have disappeared.
- Vitamin C to support your immune system. Take 3000 mg to 5000 mg per day (this is safe during breastfeeding). Split the dosage for better absorption and effect by taking 1000 mg every four hours.
- Sunflower lecithin (non-GMO) can help to thin breastmilk, making it less sticky and easier to remove from the duct. Take up to 4000 mg per day during an acute infection, splitting the dosage to 1000 mg every four hours.
- In extreme cases, antibiotics may be required.
- In cases of recurrent mastitis, we advise seeking out the support of an IBCLC, to identify the root cause and prevent it becoming an ongoing issue.

D-MER

Dysphoric Milk Ejection Reflex (D-MER) is a very rare but unpleasant phenomenon, where the breastfeeding person experiences anxiety, dread, restlessness, sadness or other negative emotions right before let-down. Very little research has been done so far, but it is thought to be related to dopamine activity associated with the milk ejection reflex. Symptoms can be mild for some, and unbearable for others. It is important to seek help from an IBCLC, who will assess the severity of your situation.

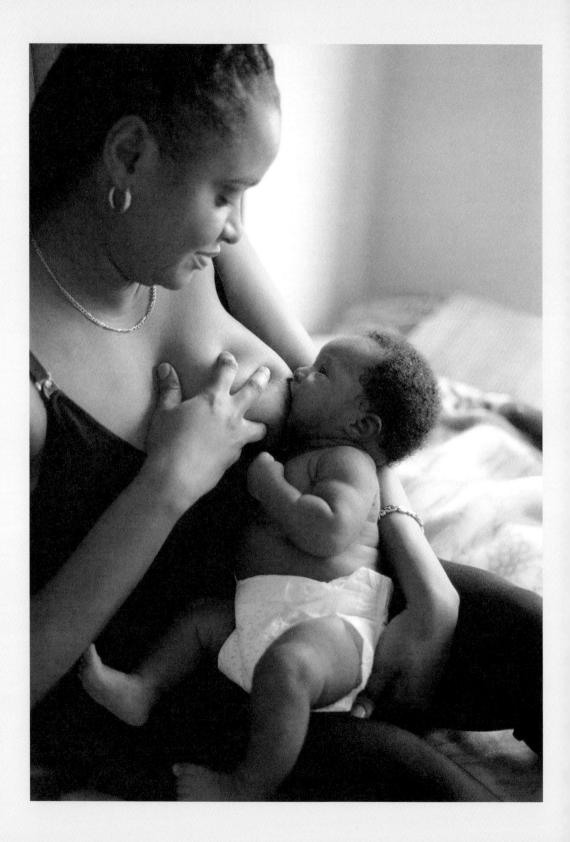

Infant Digestive Issues and Allergies

This is a HUGE topic that we simply do not have enough space to cover, and where evidence is changing rapidly.

If your baby is showing signs of reflux or colic, or you suspect they have an allergy to something in your diet, we suggest seeking out the support of an IBCLC who will help you figure out whether they are exhibiting normal infant behaviour or if there is an underlying issue that requires the support of a qualified health practitioner. An integrative doctor, naturopath or nutritionist can support you to identify and manage potential intolerances and allergies.

What About Formula?

There is no universal one-size-fits-all scenario when it comes to breastfeeding. Challenges are common no matter your circumstances and it's important to make changes if things aren't working.

As doulas, what we want every one of our readers to do is make INFORMED choices. We don't want you to quit breastfeeding if the patriarchy is making it inconvenient, but we do want you to consider making changes if your mental health is at risk.

Sometimes these changes are as simple as drinking more water, correcting your baby's latch with the help of a lactation consultant, outsourcing your food (hello meal train!), ignoring the household duties for a few days, allowing older kids to have more screen time and calling on your village. The thing is, these changes don't feel simple, because the society we live in isn't set up to support breastfeeding mothers, even though the average mother spends approximately 1800 hours breastfeeding in the first year of her child's life.

Other times, making changes simply doesn't cut it, and you may need to outsource some or all of your feeds. If breastfeeding is becoming detrimental for your mental health and you feel overwhelm, anxiety or depression creeping in, you may want to consider switching to donor or formula milk. We know many mothers who have had trouble feeding, tried donor or formula milk, and their anxieties about their babies not getting enough milk immediately melted away, resulting in an increased milk supply. Other times, introducing donor or formula milk provides huge relief and you may realise you no longer wish to breastfeed.

If you imagined yourself as a person who would feed their child until they naturally weaned, or if you've judged other people for using formula before you were in this position, you may feel conflicted.

Come back to that trick of listening to your body and leaning into your intuition. What does it say? Does the idea of breastfeeding fill you with dread, or is it something you long for? Do you feel an aversion to introducing formula, or does the idea fill you with relief? Our bodies hold all the answers. It takes work to tune into them, but they never lead us astray.

Whatever you decide, please remember that formula contains all the essential nutrients your baby needs and while it is wonderful to be able to breastfeed if you want to and are able to, what's most important is a happy and healthy baby and mother.

GALACTAGOGUES

Galacta-WHAT?

Galactagogues are foods or herbs that have been used around the world by various cultures for eons to support milk production and breastfeeding. They are often given to mothers by midwives, doulas and lactation consultants to support breastmilk supply.

The science behind how they work continues to grow. Although much of their use is based on anecdotal evidence, studies indicate their effect works on the hormonal cascade, including the increased production of prolactin, which stimulates milk production and flow.

It is important to note that galactagogues don't work to their full potential without the presence of adequate milk removal from the breast. It may also be advisable to avoid food containing galactagogues in women with oversupply. Like anything, you CAN have too much of a good thing!

Galactagogues are incredibly nutrient rich. We encourage you to combine them to create nourishing meals to enjoy on your breastfeeding journey.

Milk-Making Foods We Love:

- Oats
- Linseeds (flax seeds)
- Dark leafy greens
- Chickpeas
- Garlic
- Nettle
- Fennel seeds and bulb
- Fenugreek
- Cumin seeds
- Dill
- Nuts and nut butters
- Green papaya.

WEANING

For some, weaning comes easily and naturally, with a feed being dropped here and there until one day, you realise it's been three days since your baby asked for milk. For others, it may be a more sudden or deliberate process, hopefully taken at a pace you feel comfortable with and when you are ready for your breastfeeding relationship to end.

As you begin your weaning journey you may experience mood swings and feelings of intense sadness, anxiety and loss due to the decrease in prolactin and oxytocin associated with decreased milk production. We encourage you to be as gentle as possible with yourself during this time. Eat all the chocolate, take long baths, go for big walks in nature, or cocoon yourself in bed. Do whatever feels good so you can keep that oxytocin flowing. Remind yourself how incredible you are for nourishing your baby for as long as you did. Know that your bond will only strengthen over time, and that you will remain deeply connected to your child once breastfeeding ends. As they grow and begin to explore the world, they will always return to you – their safe space – for cuddles and connection, even if it's without a nipple in their mouth.

Some Tips to Help Create a Smooth Weaning Transition:

For You:

- Weaning tea. A blend of dried sage, peppermint and parsley will help reduce production of breastmilk.
- Do whatever you need to do to keep the oxytocin flowing! Check back on your oxytocin boosters that we listed on page 17.
- Make some artwork about breastfeeding – either alone or with your children.
- Consider getting breastmilk jewellery made.
- You may need to hand express to alleviate discomfort or engorgement. Do this in the shower. Cool packs or cabbage leaves in the bra can also help.

For Baby:

- Speak to them about the transition. If your weaning journey requires you to have a short separation from your child, and they or you are going away for a weekend, tell them that when you see them again there will be no more milk.
- Get them a special drink bottle, perhaps in their favourite colour or with their favourite characters on it. Tell them that when they want mama's milk they can drink from their special bottle instead.
- Put bandaids over your nipples so they get the visual reminder that there is no more milk.
- Wear a necklace for them to play with while they cuddle you, in place of boobs in mouth.

You may also wish to undertake a ritual together, to mark and honour the end of your breastfeeding relationship, such as baking a cake or planting a tree. While you are doing this, talk to them about your breastfeeding journey, how much you've loved it, why you are ready to stop, and thank them for breastfeeding with you.

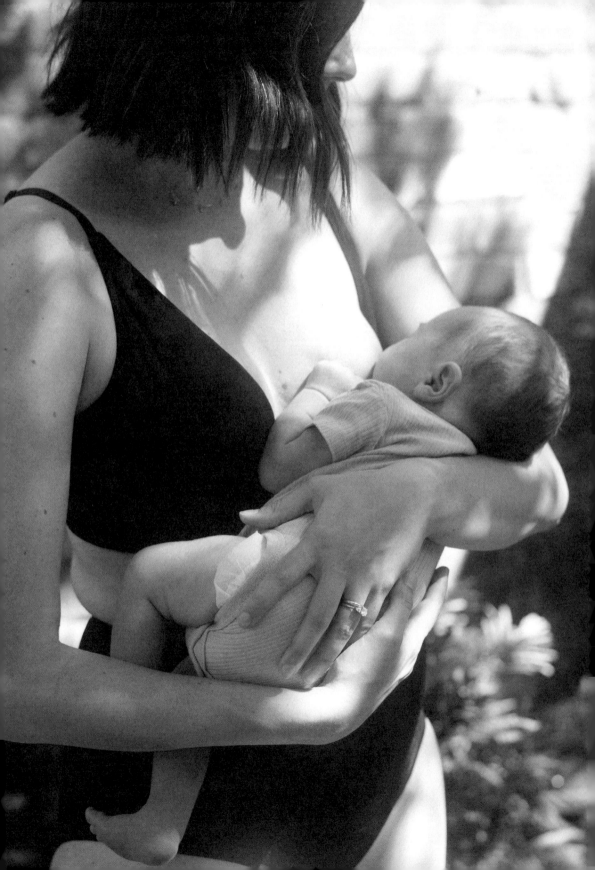

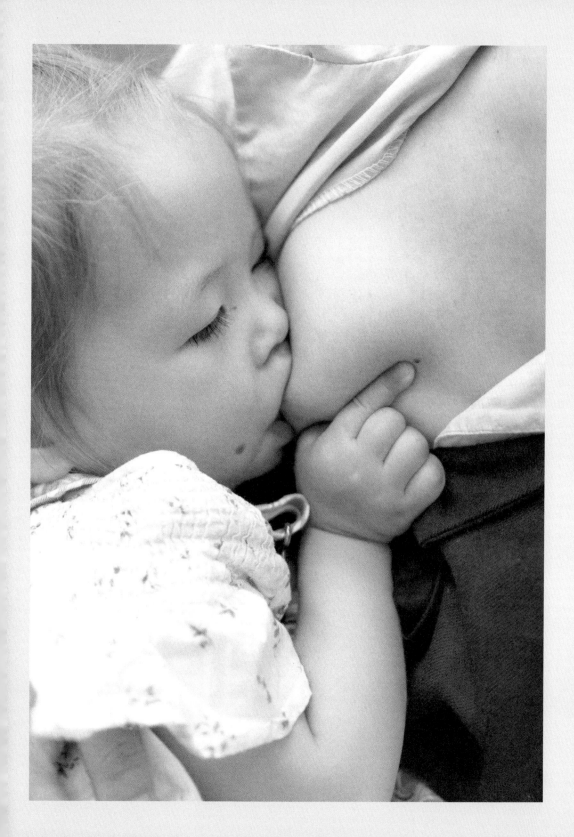

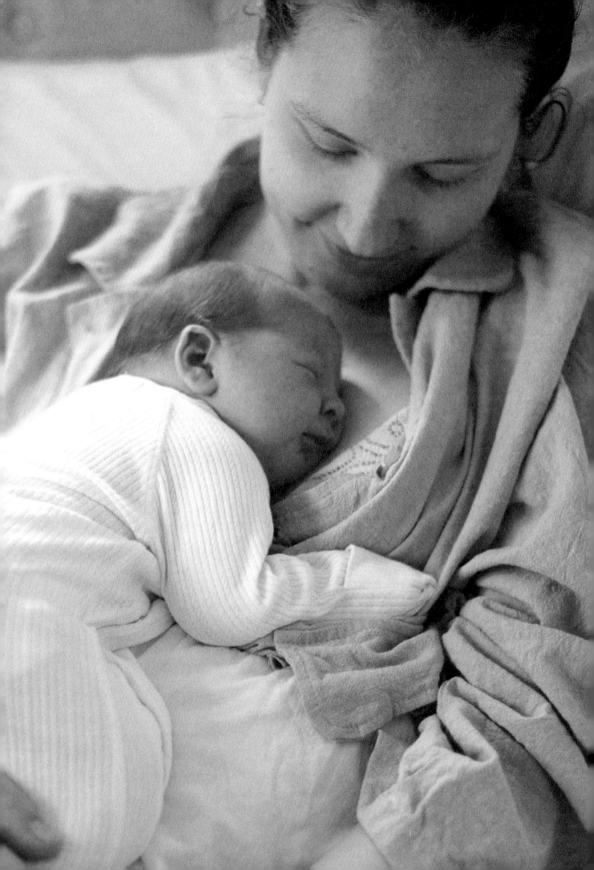

THE
FOURTH

CHAPTER THREE

TRIMESTER

Now your baby is here. What a trip, right?!

You are no doubt sore, tired, riding a tidal wave of emotions and feel as though your life has been flipped on its head. Nothing can truly prepare you for the first days at home with a newborn. Not only are you getting to know your baby, but you are also getting to know the new you, for when a baby is born, so is a mother.

The best thing you can do right now is surrender to the needs of your newborn, rest, and rest some more. For many mothers, a big hurdle to this is the accompanying guilt that comes from 'doing nothing'. Rest isn't revered in our society, but resting is the best thing you can do for you and your baby. It gives your body time to recover from the marathon of birth, it gives you space to get the hang of breastfeeding, and it allows time to bond with your precious newborn.

You may find yourself becoming restless or bored and you will likely get a burst of energy at some stage that causes you to take on more than you are capable of. This is normal and to be expected as you transition from a fast-paced life to slower, baby-led rhythms.

A wise reminder shared by Yung Pueblo in his book *Clarity & Connection*, 'Sometimes you need to move slowly so you can later move powerfully. The modern world is so fast paced that there is pressure to keep up. Setting aside what everyone else is doing and moving at your natural speed will help you make better decisions and lift your inner peace.'

'The most difficult part of birth is the first year afterwards. It is the year of travail – when the soul of a woman must birth the mother inside her. The emotional labour pains of becoming a mother are far greater than the physical pangs of birth; these are the growing surges of your heart as it pushes out selfishness and fear and makes room for sacrifice and love. It is a private and silent birth of the soul, but it is no less holy than the event of childbirth, perhaps it is even more sacred.'

JOY KUSEK

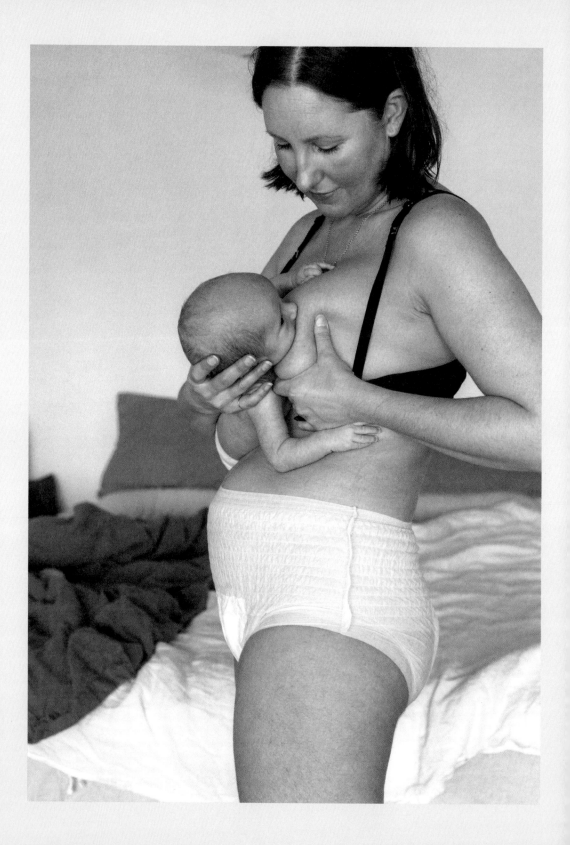

PRACTICAL BIRTH RECOVERY TIPS

Vaginal Healing

Vaginal birth comes with an onslaught of intense sensations to your nether regions in the immediate days and weeks following birth. Your vagina, vulva, perineum (the area between your vagina and anus) and rectum have had immense pressure placed upon them during the pushing or 'bearing down' stage, and a significant amount of stretching (and potentially tearing or grazing) as your baby's head and body emerged during birth.

The physical feat your body undergoes to bring your baby earthside is nothing short of a miracle, but it is also a marathon event that can leave you feeling like you just climbed the highest mountain on Earth.

It can be painful, it will be tender, it might be swollen, and that is because there is immense healing happening in every cell and fibre of your tissues and muscles as they recover and repair. Things should start to heal quite quickly, which is one of the many amazing ways that the body supports us through the physiological process of birth.

Some birthing people will be recovering from grazing, tearing, an episiotomy (an incision made in the perineum) or an instrumental birth using forceps or a vacuum. However you delivered your baby, you'll likely experience some discomfort down below for a few days or weeks. We all experience pain differently, so it is important to speak with your care provider if symptoms last longer than a few weeks, or if you feel excessive pain, discomfort, swelling or develop a fever.

Tips to Support Your Bits through Times of Discomfort:

- Ice, Ice, Baby. Using ice packs for up to a week after birth can help to reduce swelling and bruising to the vagina and perineum. After this, bringing warmth and blood flow to the area is important, which can be done using a warm pack (or bath).
- The healing power of herbs can work wonders. See recipes for Herbal Peri Pads and Herbal Healing Sitz on pages 122 and 123.
- A sitz bath is a warm, shallow bath that you sit in. It can be incredibly soothing for your nether regions and can be done in a bathtub if you have one, or using a specific 'bath' attachment for your toilet. (See recipe page 123.)
- Using a peri bottle filled with warm or cool water (depending on what feels good on the day) can help clean and soothe your perineum. Using the above Healing Herbal Sitz liquid in a peri bottle offers additional astringent, calming and antibacterial properties.
- Soak in a bath – run a warm bath and add 2 cups of Epsom salts (magnesium sulphate), which help reduce swelling and infection, and promote healing.
- If you have had an episiotomy, massage your scar when the incision is fully closed and well healed. Speak to your midwife or qualified health professional to assess when this is, so you do not break open any unhealed wounds.

Caesarean Healing

'Belly birth' involves major abdominal surgery, which can present a number of unexpected hurdles on the healing journey. Although the time it takes to meet your baby can be shorter than a vaginal birth, the hospital stay and recovery time is often longer. You will also need to go very easy on yourself, both physically and emotionally, as your internal and external incisions heal, which means giving up some physical freedoms including driving and heavy lifting in the first six weeks after birth.

During your recovery at the hospital, your care providers will monitor blood loss and signs of infection, as well as support you to get up and moving as soon as possible to prevent blood clots which are an increased risk after surgery. You should be given thorough instructions on how to care for your incision and keep yourself comfortable, which will include taking painkillers and sometimes antibiotics in the days following birth.

At the hospital and once you are home, you will experience many of the usual postpartum symptoms, including lochia and potentially 'after birth pains' as your uterus contracts and shrinks. It is important for you and your baby's wellbeing to keep yourself as comfortable as possible post-surgery, to keep the oxytocin and prolactin flowing. It's also important to note that synthetic drugs administered during a caesarean may affect how quickly your breastmilk comes in, as they can interfere with prolactin and oxytocin production.

Tips to Keep You Comfortable After a Belly Birth:

- Brace your belly. It can seriously hurt to laugh or sneeze after abdominal surgery, so keep a pillow or rolled up towel nearby to place and hold over your incision to stop your stitches feeling like they are going to pop.
- Manage your pain. You've just had major abdominal surgery and the discomfort can be overwhelming. This is not a time to be a martyr. Take the prescribed pain meds and for crying out loud, LAY THE F*CK DOWN!
- Gentle movement after surgery is important for reducing the risk of blood clots and encouraging your first postpartum poo. In the first few days, walking between rooms in your home is well and truly enough. As you gain strength, small and gentle excursions outside may feel manageable. Don't overdo it. A simple walk around the block is more than enough for the first few weeks postpartum.
- Ask for help. Again, this is not a time to be a martyr. If you know someone who has undergone major surgery, you know how much assistance and support is needed while they recover. A caesarean is no exception and asking for help will allow you to rest, heal and bond with your baby.
- Blood loss during a caesarean is approximately two times more than a vaginal birth, so ensure to eat plenty of collagen, iron and vitamin C rich foods to boost your iron stores and encourage healing and repair of your skin, tissues and muscles.
- Massage your scar when the incision is fully closed and well healed. Speak to your midwife or other qualified health professional to assess when it is safe to do so.

Haemorrhoids

Haemorrhoids are swollen veins in or around your anus, which are incredibly common during pregnancy and postpartum, most often after a vaginal birth. These can be found internally (generally painless) and externally (often painful), and can be caused by the prolonged strain of constipation and pressure placed on the veins in your rectum during pregnancy and labour. Symptoms include itchiness, pain, bleeding after pooing (often seen on toilet paper when you wipe) and swelling in and around your anus.

Haemorrhoids can shrink and disappear with the correct support. Here are some gentle ways to avoid and reduce them:

- Eat fibre-rich foods including vegetables, fruits and whole grains. These help to bulk and soften your stool, which reduces your need to strain when pooing.
- Hydrate! Drink plenty of water and herbal tea throughout the day to help to soften your stool.
- Witch-hazel distillate (alcohol free) is an anti-inflammatory astringent, which helps to reduce pain and swelling of haemorrhoids. Soak a cotton pad with the liquid and apply directly to your haemorrhoids after each bowel movement. Do this several times per day and keep your witch-hazel in the fridge so it feels extra cool and soothing.
- Soaking in a sitz bath for 15 minutes after you poo can be incredibly soothing. Do it up to three times a day and add 1 cup of Epsom salts for additional therapeutic benefits.
- Avoid low-fibre foods that slow down your digestive system, including white bread, chips, baked goods and sugary treats.

Anal Fissures

Anal fissures sound intense but they are quite common. They present as painful cuts or tears around the anus (similar to a cracked lip) and are often caused by constipation or chronic diarrhoea, or the trauma of pressure placed on the rectum during birth. Symptoms are similar to haemorrhoids, however pain is often most common following a bowel movement. Anal fissures often heal within four to six weeks if cared for correctly. Most of the recommendations for haemorrhoids are suitable for anal fissures, however you should not use witch-hazel or any other astringent, alcohol-based wipes as they will sting.

Diastasis Recti

Diastasis recti, commonly known as abdominal separation, affects more than 50 per cent of new mothers in the postpartum. During pregnancy, the connective tissue that supports your rectus abdominis (six pack muscles) thins and stretches to accommodate your growing baby and stretching uterus. This is a normal process of pregnancy, and smaller separations will often resolve naturally within the first two months after birth. In larger separations, women often notice a bulge between their abdominal muscles when lifting their child or sitting up from a lying position. When cases are severe or left untreated, diastasis recti can cause back pain, poor posture, pelvic floor instability, bloating, hernia and pain during sex. It is important to have any concerns assessed by a qualified pelvic floor physiotherapist, so they can create a recovery plan for you. Recovery usually takes three to six months depending on the degree of separation and other contributing factors.

BLOOD, SWEAT AND TEARS

There Will Be Blood

Remember when we told you to buy adult diapers in the first chapter?

In the days following birth, your uterus releases an unfathomable amount of blood and gunk (mucus, amniotic fluid and uterine tissue), commonly known as lochia. This bleeding may be accompanied by pain as your uterus contracts (commonly known as 'after-birth pains'), especially while breastfeeding, as breastfeeding hormones stimulate the uterus to return to its pre-baby size. It is also normal to pass blood clots, however anything larger than a golf ball should be flagged with your care provider, as should excessive bleeding or unusual smells, which can be signs of infection.

Heavy lochia will generally last up to five days, after which you should find it light enough to switch to pads or period undies. It's important to note that nothing should be inserted into your vagina for the first six weeks following birth (including period cups, tampons, penises or sex toys), regardless of whether you birthed vaginally or via caesarean, as these may cause infection.

General bleeding may last for up to six weeks as the placental wound heals, and you may find it ebbs and flows, or starts and stops several times. It is common to experience heavy bleeding after spending too much time on your feet; this is your body's way of telling you to get horizontal and rest.

There Will Be Sweat

One of the most surprising things during the postpartum may be the profuse amount of sweat you produce. During pregnancy, your blood volume increases significantly, which requires an increase in water retention. After birth, the hormones that caused your body to hold onto water during pregnancy are now telling your body to flush the excess fluid out. This naturally occurs through your skin, often during the night, where you may find yourself waking up drenched. You'll hear us talking about hydration a lot throughout this book, and this is one of the reasons why. Drinking plenty of water not only supports your body during this process, but also encourages you to urinate any excess liquid, rather than sweat it out.

If you are breastfeeding, you may also find your underarms emit a stronger odour than usual. This is your body's way of ensuring that your baby can find its food source (you!). Cool, right?!

Tips to Support Your Sweats:

- Sleep on towels to prevent a middle of the night sheet change
- Take a warm or cool shower in the morning
- Consume plenty of hydrating fluids (water and herbal teas)
- Wear clothing made from natural, breathable fibres (cotton, bamboo, linen)
- Open doors and windows for fresh air
- Hang tight, this should only last a few weeks.

There Will Be Sh!t (and P!ss)

The first postpartum poo can be utterly terrifying.

Those of you who birthed vaginally have had your nether regions stretched beyond their wildest imagination. Even if you didn't require stitches, you probably feel bruised and sore in your rectal and perineal area and are likely to be sporting haemorrhoids. You also may not have had a bowel movement for a week, and things might be feeling pretty clogged up. This physiological shift occurs as your digestive system and hormones re-regulate, and is also a very common side effect from being administered pharmaceutical drugs during labour, which can interfere with and slow down bowel function. Naturally, this also applies to those of you who gave birth via caesarean.

Tips for Bathroom Trips:

- Eat plenty of fibre-rich foods, including fresh fruit and cooked vegetables (preferably with skin on, as they contain insoluble fibre which helps to bulk and soften your poo to make it easier to pass). Other poo-friendly sources of fibre include: chia and linseeds (flax seeds), psyllium husk and slippery elm (which must be taken with sufficient water, or they can exacerbate the issue). Porridge topped with our Spiced Digestive Compote (page 191) is an excellent way to get things going.
- HYDRATE! Lubricating your digestive system with good old H2O helps to rehydrate your colon. This will help soften your stool and allow you to pass it more easily. It will also encourage frequent urination which is important for reducing the risk of urinary tract infections (UTIs).
- Focus on relaxing your pelvic floor to help relax your bowels and bladder. If you are having trouble, flag this with your care provider. A pelvic floor physio or specialist is highly recommended. (This also applies if you are experiencing urinary or faecal incontinence.)
- Elevate your feet using a low stool or a roll of toilet paper under each foot. This shifts you into prime pooing position, enabling things to move with ease.
- Using clean hands or a pad, apply light pressure to your perineum while pooing and gently breathe the poo out, just like when you are in labour. Avoid straining as this can create or worsen haemorrhoids. If you have a caesarean wound, use a rolled-up towel and apply light pressure to support stitches and abdominal muscles.
- Use a peri bottle or hand bidet filled with warm, salty water after you poo as a gentle way of cleansing your perineum and anus, especially if you have haemorrhoids which can be difficult to clean. Pat dry with a clean towel afterwards.
- Consider taking digestive enzymes, to help your stomach break down food and digest essential nutrients, as well as magnesium citrate, which attracts water to the colon and supports bowel movements.
- Urinating can sting like a motherf*cker, due to grazes, stitches and tearing that can take several weeks to heal. Using a peri bottle to squirt warm water on the affected area while urinating can work wonders at reducing the discomfort.

There Will Be Tears

Vaughne's personal hero Aviva Romm says, 'The postpartum hormone drop is considered the single largest sudden hormone change in the shortest amount of time for any human being, at any point of their life cycle.'

During pregnancy, our oestrogen and progesterone skyrocket to levels never experienced before. During labour, our body produces a cocktail of hormones (hello adrenaline and oxytocin) which come crashing down afterwards. Add a surge in prolactin to help you create breastmilk and not surprisingly, around days three to five postpartum, you may experience something like PMS on steroids (or if your 20s were anything like ours, a post-party comedown), commonly known as the 'baby blues'.

This can be accompanied by huge emotional changes. Many birthing people find themselves weepy and anxious, wondering if there is something wrong with them, as their body processes this hormonal drop. Even those who know it is coming may need a reminder that what they are feeling is completely normal.

Tips for Your Tears:

- Know that it is normal and that it will pass. 'This too shall pass' is an excellent mantra to keep in mind for difficult times in motherhood. If you experience overwhelming or prolonged feelings of sadness or anxiety, reach out to a qualified health professional.
- Sharing your thoughts and feelings with someone you trust (and who won't trivialise what you are going through) will help you move through negative emotions more quickly.
- Watch or listen to things that make you cry happy tears. Happy tears and sad tears produce different hormones, however a big emotional release is sometimes all we need to help us feel balanced again.
- Refer back to your list of oxytocin boosters on page 17. These will be different for everyone as we all have different pick-me-ups.
- Flower essences. We think Rescue Remedy is brilliant. Our business Mama Goodness has created a blend of flower essences named Zen Drops, which is like Rescue Remedy, but with the specific needs of mums in mind. We ship internationally, but you can also look for a blend by Alexis Smart or if you have access to a naturopath, ask them to make you a blend.

Your Baby Will Cry Too

In the words of Abi Davis and Robin Kramer, 'Children do not have the necessary language skills to communicate their pain, hunger, or discomfort. Instead, they cry.'

Society may have conditioned you to think that you're supposed to know what your baby's cries mean and it can be disheartening when you can't decipher them. We've got to let you in on a little secret – most other parents don't know either, at least not in the beginning.

'Needs crying' is when babies cry to communicate that they are unhappy about something. It may be hunger, thirst, tiredness, a dirty nappy, the need for a cuddle, they might be too hot, too cold, or it might even be the case of that adorable outfit being really uncomfortable.

Most 'needs cries' can be amended with a quick once-over of the things listed above. When that doesn't work, they may simply be in need of a 'release cry', in which case, the best thing you can do is hold them close and let them cry.

'Release crying' is when babies cry to release tension. Remember, babies pick up on absolutely everything that's going on around them, including how you feel. Safe in your loving arms, they cry to release the overwhelm of the day, which can be due to overstimulation, taking on our emotions, or even because they need to process birth trauma. Many babies exhibit fussiness, irritability and crying between the hours of 4 pm and 11 pm, which has been dubbed the 'witching hour'. Extended crying can completely unravel even the most calm caregiver, and can feel like a cruel catch-22 because in order for them to feel calm they need us to feel calm, but it is really f*cking hard to stay calm when your baby won't stop crying.

While popping them in a pram and going for a walk around the block may seem like a good idea and a way to reset, when they are in need of a release cry, this will likely lead to more overstimulation. Being in the safety of your arms – skin-to-skin if possible – and in a quiet, dark room where they feel safe, is the best way to help them move through what is upsetting them and return to a peaceful state. Talk to them, tell them you know they've had a hard day and it's okay, you're here now and they are safe with you and they can let it out. If you feel overwhelmed when your baby cries, ear plugs can help reduce the volume while you tend to them. If retreating to a room or holding them for hours on end is not an option, popping them in a carrier will hold them close while giving you the freedom to tend to other children or household tasks.

While a crying baby usually wants to be in the arms of a loving caregiver, shaking a baby can cause serious and irreversible brain damage, and even death. If you feel triggered by relentless crying and feel anger or frustration rising within you, it is safer to hand them to your partner or lay them down in a safe place and walk away. Take some deep breaths and try to find your calm. Have a glass of ice-cold water, phone a friend if you need to, then return to your baby when you feel calm.

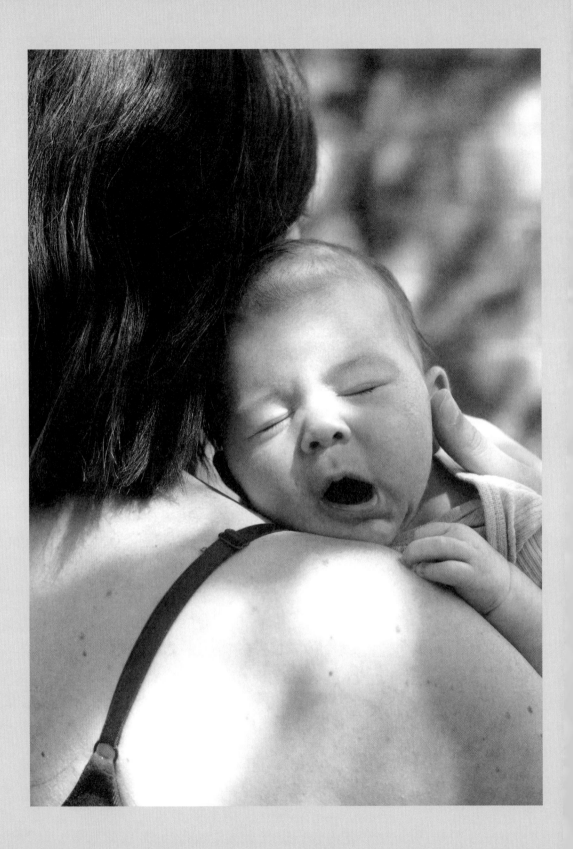

MENTAL HEALTH AND OTHER BIG FEELS

Studies show that one in four mothers will experience high levels of depressive symptoms in the first three years after giving birth, with postpartum depression most commonly being diagnosed when the firstborn child is four years old. These statistics are alarming and bring awareness to the ongoing needs of mothers, who need to be assessed and supported long after the current routine six-week or six-month check-in with general practitioners.

Why? Because the undertaking of parenthood is no easy feat. Without doubt, becoming a parent can be the most fulfilling, positively life altering, beautiful experience in the world, but it is also a huge, all-encompassing undertaking of the mind, body and soul. For some, the nights will be long, the days will be boring and exhaustion will make you question your sanity, but the intense love for your child and being in their presence every day will make it worthwhile. For others, it will be the hardest thing you have ever done and motherhood will feel like it has swallowed you whole, triggering thoughts of running away for a night or three (or forever).

There is no right or wrong way to feel; motherhood is an experience so individual that no one will ever truly know how deep and dark your thoughts can go at 3 am with a baby glued to your chest. But there is a huge amount of information to support and guide you through the kaleidoscope of emotions and moods. You are never alone and every mood disorder we mention in this section is both temporary and treatable. Sharing your feelings with people you trust and seeking support from health professionals takes courage, but it is the first step in getting the help you so greatly deserve.

So what do you need to look out for?

Baby Blues

The baby blues can be a shock to any new mother in the first few days and weeks after birth. They are commonly experienced by new mothers and are a natural adjustment that occurs when faced with the dramatic hormonal shift after birth, as well as the initial, often stressful adjustment to life with a new baby. Between 50 to 80 per cent of new mothers report feeling symptoms including sadness, irritation and exhaustion. However, if these feelings continue to affect you after the first month of motherhood and interfere with your ability to function or parent, you might be experiencing something more serious like Perinatal Mood and Anxiety Disorders (PMADs).

Perinatal Mood and Anxiety Disorders (PMADs)

PMADs are a group of symptoms that can occur during pregnancy and postpartum, and can cause both emotional and physical distress that disrupt a mother's outlook and ability to function. Below are the different types of PMADs.

POSTPARTUM DEPRESSION (PPD)

Experienced beyond the first month of parenthood, postpartum depression may be characterised by:

- Apathy, sadness or tearfulness
- Anger or rage
- Loss of or increase in appetite
- Absence of joy
- Low energy
- Insomnia
- Difficulty concentrating
- Feelings of guilt or shame
- Thoughts of harming yourself or your baby.

More than 15 per cent of birthing people are said to experience PPD, with suicide being the leading cause of maternal death in the first year of a child's life.

Remember, every case of postpartum depression is different and you don't need to have all the symptoms. It is common to resist the idea that you are struggling mentally, especially if you haven't had mental health struggles in the past. If you are struggling, please seek help. No matter what your brain is telling you, your family is NOT better off without you. They also may not understand what is going on for you, unless you voice it. If you don't feel comfortable sharing how you are feeling with someone in your immediate care circle, please, PLEASE call a mental health support line. Many countries have a helpline that is specifically for maternal mental health support.

It is important to note that PPD can also affect dads. While symptoms may be similar to those with maternal PPD, studies show that paternal PPD may manifest in different ways such as aggression, substance abuse and hypersexuality.

POSTPARTUM ANXIETY

Many new mothers feel they have a thousand things to worry about after having a baby. If your anxiety is interfering with your overall functioning, you may be experiencing postpartum anxiety. Postpartum anxiety may be characterised by:

- Incessant worrying, catastrophising or panic
- Inability to switch off
- Loss of or increase in appetite
- Sleep disturbances
- Chest tightness, nausea, dizziness, racing heart and other physical symptoms.

Like most of the PMADS, postpartum anxiety is common with one in every ten people experiencing symptoms in the first year following birth. As with postpartum depression, there are hotlines in most parts of the world that you can call when you are spiralling or need immediate support. We highly recommend seeking out a mental health practitioner to support you on an ongoing basis.

POSTPARTUM PSYCHOSIS

While rare, postpartum psychosis is a serious condition that requires immediate medical attention. It may be characterised by:

- Delusions or hallucinations
- Paranoia and suspiciousness
- Confusion or disorientation
- Disconnection from others and reality
- Agitation or extreme mood swings
- Insomnia or decreased need for sleep.

While postpartum psychosis affects less than 0.2 per cent of all birthing people and although acts of harm to oneself or the baby are uncommon, it may cause erratic behaviours and place you and your family in danger. People suffering from postpartum psychosis often don't realise they are having an episode. It is therefore important for everyone in your support circle to be aware of the symptoms so they can seek urgent medical attention if required.

POSTPARTUM OCD

Postpartum OCD is characterised by intrusive thoughts regarding the wellbeing of your baby and subsequent compulsive behaviours.

- Intrusive thoughts or obsessions are persistent and irrational thoughts or mental images, often macabre and upsetting in nature.
- Compulsions are repetitive behaviours to try and prevent those fears and obsessions from happening.

Postpartum OCD can affect 3 to 5 per cent of people and may leave you with a sense of horror, fear of being left alone with your baby, and hypervigilance in protecting them, for example constantly checking on them as they sleep, or constantly cleaning.

Many mothers who experience these symptoms are aware their thoughts are strange, therefore the likelihood of acting on or following through is low.

Side note: Some people may experience intrusive thoughts without developing OCD. While unpleasant, it is important to note this is normal. We are biologically hardwired to protect our babies and it is natural to imagine that harm may come to your baby. While not commonly acknowledged by general practitioners and the maternal care community, intrusive thoughts affect many, many mothers and parents. Before knowing that they are normal, intrusive thoughts may have you feeling concerned, however sometimes the simple act of putting a name to it is enough to help you understand what is happening.

Anger and Rage

We live in a society where anger is vilified and thus it is often shut down, ignored, contained or concealed, however anger is almost always related to an unmet need. When we reframe our perception of anger as a signal that something isn't right or something needs to change, we can use it as a guiding force. It may be telling us to find new ways of doing things, or it might be helping us identify sources of unhealed trauma that need healing.

Feelings of rage, resentment, anger, overwhelm, being touched out or losing control can be scary, but they are more common than you may think. It is important to understand that these intense feelings are normal to a degree, however if you feel that you are frequently losing control, you may wish to speak with a trusted care provider and learn some coping mechanisms. Remember – your emotions are a signal that something isn't working. Identifying what needs to change can be incredibly beneficial to the wellbeing of your entire family, as can learning to regulate your emotions – as discussed on page 23.

Tips for when you're feeling out of control:

1. Isolate from your baby (e.g. pop them in their bassinet).
2. Take deep, slow breaths. Breathe in for five seconds and out for five seconds. Do this five times.
3. Splash your face with cold water.
4. If you cannot calm yourself, call a safe person who you can talk with to help calm you down.

As your children grow older, you may find that rage is something you experience often. Many, many mothers in our community report going from zero to 100 over something seemingly minor, which is especially surprising to those who have never experienced anger or rage in the past. Because anger is almost always related to an unmet need, it is important to lean on the support of your village and carve out time for yourself to ensure that your own needs are being met. When you parent from a resourced place, you are less likely to feel overwhelmed when others constantly need you. You absolutely cannot wait for others to do this for you, because no one understands your needs as intrinsically as you do.

Phantom Crying:

Phantom crying is when you think you hear your baby crying but they aren't. This is common when they are napping and you are doing something noisy such as taking a shower or vacuuming. While it's not linked to mental health, it can make you wonder if you are losing your mind, so we wanted to note it here as a common phenomenon.

The Importance of Sharing Our Birth Stories

BY KIMBERLY ANN JOHNSON, FROM *THE FOURTH TRIMESTER*

Our dominant cultural narrative is that so long as mother and baby survive the birth experience and are relatively healthy by Western medicine standards, the birth was successful. This discounts many women's experiences. Even though yes, they are healthy and yes, their baby is healthy, their bodies, minds and souls are still deeply affected. Like so much of the way our culture works, the process itself is exchanged for the outcome, in this case the birth experience is discounted because you have a healthy baby.

While giving birth there are pivotal moments where we must face ourselves at deeper levels, where we come face-to-face with unexpected obstacles or unanticipated reservoirs of strength. When we reduce the experience to the outcome – and specifically to the rote idea that so long as a woman is alive, everything went well – we overlook an untapped resource. The woman and her community miss out on a chance to gain wisdom and maturity from her experience.

As you contemplate your birth experience, notice how your body feels. Tell your story from your heart, paying attention to the sensations in your body. It is not important to remember every detail in perfect order but rather, to document significant moments and how you felt during them.

When your partner shares his or her experience of the birth, you may be surprised to hear a version that is different from yours. Your partner may have memories of moments you don't recall at all. What seemed important to you may not have seemed at all important to him. What is important is listening to each other without arguing over the details, and without any needs to change, fix or convince. Listen for the moments that are turning points. Listen for the places that your partner repeats themselves, gets emphatic, or changes the volume of their voice as clues to what may have been exhilarating or scary for them.

Oftentimes, it takes a couple of rounds of telling our stories over time to find the meaning they have for us. We may feel confounded by something our partner is hanging onto that felt insignificant for us. Our partner may not understand why we cannot move past or get over parts of the birth that seemed necessary, normal, and even practical to them. We don't actually have to understand, we just have to listen wholeheartedly.

Our stories evolve over time and that is healthy. When a narrative never changes, we are not growing or developing our ability to see the meaning of our stories in deepening layers. With an experience as big as giving birth and becoming parents, it may take time to find a way forward with a joint narrative that honours each other's experiences and to make the repairs necessary for healing.

Whether we tell our story by writing it, speaking it, recording it or making art with it, there will be power in telling your birth story. You may find critical pieces of self-understanding and understanding of your mother–child bond or your partner bond in the process. You may find that the ways you look at yourself are influenced by specific statements or circumstances from the birth. It is often the births where something needs healing whose story needs to be told.

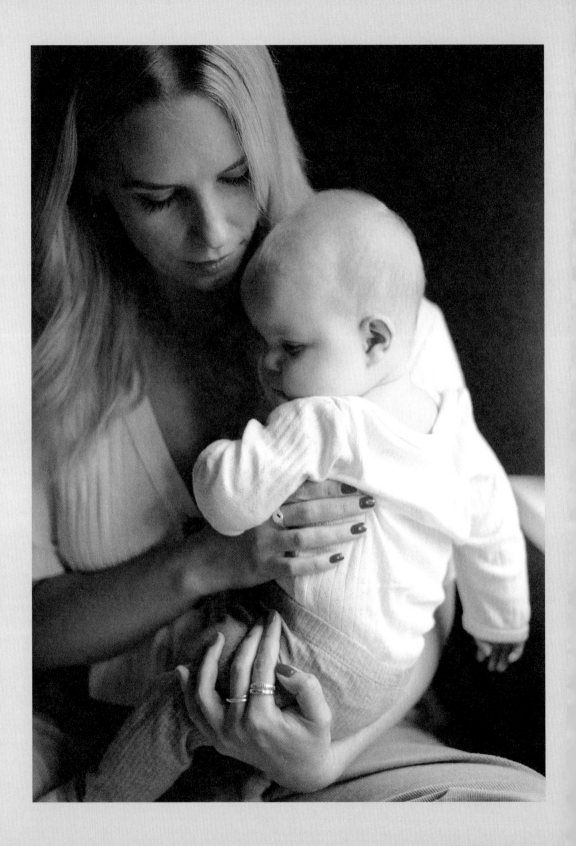

UNCONVENTIONAL POSTPARTUM

We cannot write a book on the postpartum without honouring those who will not bring their baby home whether that be due to health complications and extended time spent at the hospital, or due to the heartbreaking reality of loss.

Neonatal Intensive Care Unit (NICU) Parents

Vaughne's first doula client was serendipitously her best friend, Aimee, who she was lucky enough to live with through the majority of her pregnancy, as well as support through the heartbreaking news that her daughter Edie, while in utero, was suffering from a health issue that would require immediate care in the NICU following birth. Aimee and Edie spent eight long months of their first year together at Melbourne's Royal Children's Hospital, navigating daily assessments, weekly procedures and four major surgeries undertaken by incredible doctors and nurses who saved Edie's life.

Navigating the trauma and grief of a sick baby, on top of juggling the physical and emotional load that all new mothers deal with, is an enormous, all-consuming and terrifying roller-coaster for any new parent. The news of a stay in NICU, no matter how long, can come before or after birth and turn any parent's world completely inside out and upside down.

Below, Aimee offers her insights and suggestions for other parents who will experience having a child in NICU.

- Accept help and support such as meal deliveries, people bringing you fresh clothes and toiletries, looking after other children, pets or housework, or coming to the hospital to visit if you are feeling up for it.
- Remember to eat and drink – it can be a blur inside some days, but you need to be nourished so that you can have energy, both physically and emotionally, to be there for your child.
- Take time to get some fresh air. As much as you feel uncomfortable leaving, go for a gentle walk or sit outside at least once a day. It might feel terrifying to leave the hospital room but taking care of yourself is important to avoid getting run down or sick. It will make a difference, I promise.
- Life in hospital can be isolating and lonely. When you feel ready, connect with other NICU parents. When friends or family continue to go about their lives, finding other parents with a shared experience can be soothing and bring a sense of community and acceptance. Hang on to each other gently, one day at a time.
- If you make parent friends, be prepared to watch them leave with their baby before you do. This can be a hard pill to swallow. Even though it's wonderful for them, it's okay to feel angry, bitter and sad that it's not you leaving.
- You will likely experience residual trauma and a kaleidoscope of emotions ranging from despair to anger to dissociation. Seek professional help. Social workers are often available to support you through the difficult times. The hospital may or may not offer counselling or psychology services, but for your own wellbeing and long-term recovery, please seek the guidance and support of a mental health professional during your stay at the hospital, and once you return home.

Miscarriage, Infant Loss and Abortion

As doulas, we have come to understand and honour the truth that birth and death cannot exist without each other. For many on the beautiful and brutal journey of motherhood, there exists a commonly shared but under acknowledged experience of loss.

One in five pregnancies will end due to miscarriage during the first trimester, while close to 1 per cent of babies will be stillborn or die in the first month of life, leaving parents adrift and left to grapple with confusion, heartbreak and grief. In Australia, an additional one in four women will choose to have an abortion. Common feelings experienced following a miscarriage, stillbirth, abortion or termination for medical reasons (TFMR) may include sadness, anger, numbness, shame, guilt, jealousy and embarrassment.

It is important to recognise that no matter what an individual's experience or choice was in the loss of their child, once a woman has carried a foetus in their womb, they are forever in their postpartum. Cellular changes occur in the body and brain following conception that remain forever. This is why we believe society should revere, show empathy for, grieve with, and support women through this loss.

Loss can be a tumultuous process of grief, recovery and healing for many women and this should not be rushed or overlooked. Physical and emotional recovery is unique to every individual and takes time, softness for yourself and your body, as well as the support of trusted friends, family and community.

There is no single way to process loss, however there are some beautifully nurturing tools to support your body and mind as you navigate your own experience.

Loss is hard on your heart and body. Cramping and contractions can range from mild to severe and blood loss can be significant over the course of several days. Breastmilk may also begin to flow. Other symptoms may include headaches, nausea and intense emotions, all of which can deplete your resolve.

REST

Your body is going through an immense recalibration on both an emotional and physical level. This is not a time to continue with the fast-paced way of living that society generally demands from us, but, rather, a time to heal and replenish. It is important to create a comfortable environment that allows you to remain in bed or on the couch, and to have uninterrupted sleep when you feel like it. We also recommend you avoid strenuous activities and high intensity exercise as you allow your body to heal. If your nervous system is craving movement, lean into gentle exercise including walking, stretching and yoga.

NOURISH YOURSELF

Nourishing your body with nutrient dense, quality wholefoods is important when recovering from loss. When you experience physical or emotional pain it is best to avoid refined sugar, processed carbs and alcohol, as these can increase inflammation and discomfort and heighten emotions. Instead, focus on eating traditional postpartum foods that will help your body heal and repair because you are in your postpartum too.

EMOTIONAL SUPPORT

Historically, our culture is blind to the enormity of loss. It often takes a long time to recover from the experience, while leaving many women and their partners emotionally fragile. We experience a multitude of emotions while grieving that are not always expected and that is okay. People have very different experiences when it comes to grief and although experts outline the stages of grief, these are guidelines and not a 'textbook' response.

Asking for support from your partner, family and friends may feel uncomfortable but is exactly what you need and will create a loving nest around you. People often feel relieved and enthusiastic to provide comfort and practical support, so allow yourself to be cared for during a time that you need it the most.

Tips for navigating the emotions of loss:

- Allow yourself and your partner time to move through the waves of emotions and process your loss.
- Share your feelings with your partner and invite them to do the same. It's important and validating, and encourages you both to reflect and connect.
- Sharing your feelings and experience with people you trust can be healing and help you make meaning from your loss. Seek support from family, friends or health professionals who offer non-judgemental, sound, safe and informed advice and perspective. This may include your midwife, doula, doctor, counsellor or psychologist.
- Seek organisations that offer guidance and support through all stages of pregnancy and postpartum. Two great resources are:
  - **The Pink Elephants:** *www.pinkelephants.org.au*
  - **SANDS:** *www.sands.org.au*
- Hold a loving ceremony to say goodbye to your baby. Light candles, build a fire, read or burn a letter you have written, plant seeds or a tree in their honour or release flowers into the ocean.

How to Support Perinatal Grief and Loss

BY LILLY LOWREY

Lilly Lowrey is a fellow doula and perinatal mental health professional, who has shared some practical and emotional ways to support those going through the heartbreak of loss. It may be handy to reference if anyone you know ever experiences loss, and may be helpful to share with loved ones if you yourself ever experience loss.

Non-judgemental, compassionate space holding is the foundation of companioning someone who has experienced perinatal loss – which encompasses miscarriage, abortion, stillbirth and the loss of a newborn. While most of us want to show up in a meaningful way for the people we love, we might also feel awkward, unsure and anxious about what is the 'right thing' to say or do.

As support people it's important to remember that what we say, and what we don't say, can deeply affect someone who is grieving. So, where can we start and what does 'holding space' look like?

'Holding space' simply means being wholeheartedly present for someone. When we hold space for someone who is grieving, we acknowledge and witness that person as they are in that moment without trying to 'fix' them. By being present – emotionally, physically and mentally – we are creating a safe space for them to share their story without judgement, to be held in loving support, and to feel less alone.

Although nothing we say can take away from what the person is feeling – whether that be grief, sadness, guilt or anger – acknowledging their loss and offering validating statements can provide solidarity. Always offer support from a place of compassion and be authentic. If you know someone who has lost their baby, ask how they are feeling and acknowledge the loss even if it feels awkward. This will mean more to them than you will ever know.

Some examples of validating statements are:

'I am so sorry for your loss of baby _____. My heart is with you.'
'Your feelings are valid. Take your time and be gentle with yourself along the way.'
'I know these last few months have been really hard. I'm proud of you for getting through.'
'It's okay to take your time, you deserve patience. I'm always here for you.'

And while thoughtful words can offer acknowledgment and validation, when we are fully present with someone who is grieving, silence can also be medicine. Your physical presence, a warm hug, or a tender look can offer comfort.

Lastly, remember that grief after loss is complex, messy and multifaceted. And while there are common threads, it is deeply personal and will look different for everyone. Grief is not a linear process, nor does it move through predictable stages. We are human beings, not machines. So, keep showing up for the people you love. Offer open-ended support. Really see them, hold them, and honour their grief as a journey.

Doin' It Solo

BY CATIE GETT

While everything we share in this book is applicable to all birthing people, we realise some don't have that support person, extra pair of hands and someone to bear witness to it all – the beautiful, the messy, the mundane, and to say, 'You're doing an amazing job!'

You don't need us telling you how to solo parent, but naturopath, author and solo mum Catie Gett shares some ways you can ask your community to assist – it may be worth taking a photo of this list and sharing it with friends and family.

While no two families are the same, if you're doing it solo, it's easy to feel like there is no family like yours. The decision to raise a family on your own is never made lightly and may even have been unexpected.

Social constructs can make women feel like failures if they do not have a partner, but single parents are not failures. This culture is broken and outdated.

This list is a collection of the things that my loved ones did for me, but it is also a list of things I wish they had known to do. I wrote it laughing while letting the tears run down my face. It brought up the times when I thought loneliness would swallow me whole and when tiredness was so deep in my bones I thought I would never re-emerge as myself ever again.

'To-Do' list for the solo parents in your life:

- If you are on the way to their home check to see if they need anything from the shops. When you get there, do the dishes, read their child/ren a book, weed the garden.
- Take photos of them with their child/ren.
- Love their child/ren. Let them tell you stories and shower you with photos. This will make it less isolating for them.
- Tell them they are a really good parent.
- Keep inviting them to things no matter how many times they say no.
- Take their child/ren to buy a mother's/father's day gift or help them make a card.
- Check in with them if/when their child/ren go to the other parent's house. This is often a really difficult time, especially in the beginning.
- Don't say 'the break must be good'. For many parents it can feel like their child/ren have been taken from them each time they visit their other parent.
- Engage with their child/ren. Be a safe person for their child so they have moments to breathe.
- Help with day-to-day logistics like picking the child/ren up from school.
- Have them as part of your family, invite them on family outings and holidays.
- Give them a social life that fits their lifestyle, like popping over with a bottle of wine after the child/ren are asleep.
- Listen to them. Some days you may be the only adult they have spoken to.
- Before offering advice, ask 'how and where can I turn up for you?'
- Help them remember they are more than just a parent.
- Don't ever complain to them about being tired.
- Remember that just because they're carrying it all, doesn't mean it's not heavy.

To those of you that are new single parents and to those that may become one soon: I know that right now is scary and isolating, but I promise you the best days of your life are ahead. You and your children will share a magical bond. The greatest paradox of solo parenthood is that while it is a logistical circus, it is also beautifully simple.

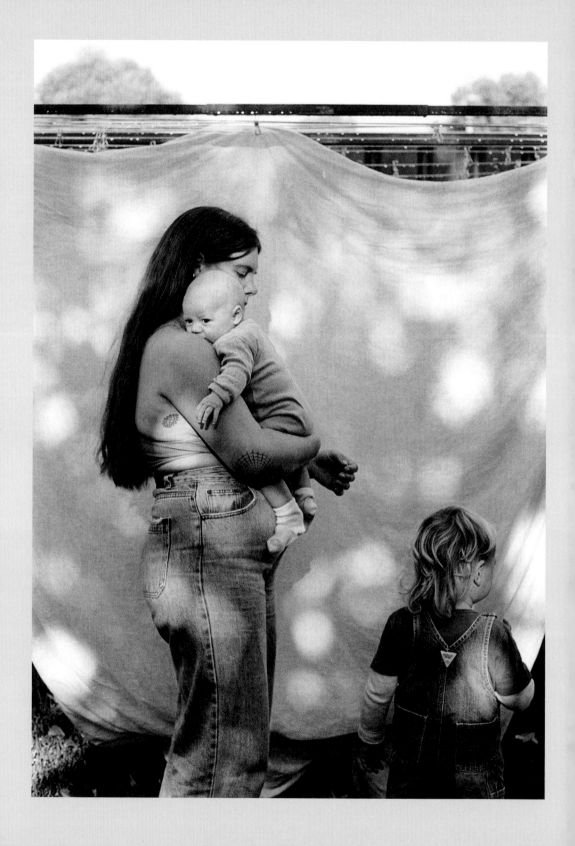

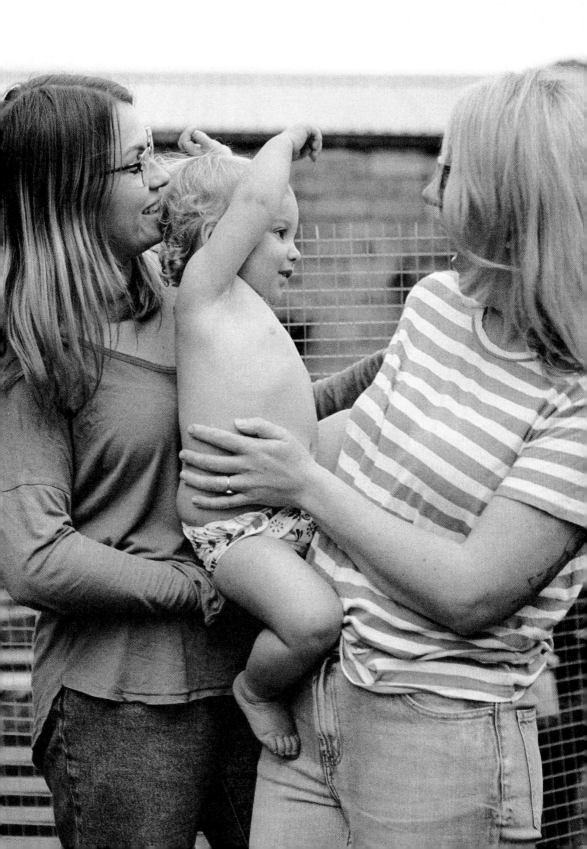

Your Pelvic Floor

BY KAITLYN BYWATER

Kaitlyn Bywater is a musculoskeletal physiotherapist and mother to three boys. Saddened at the lack of pelvic floor care afforded to birthing people, she is on a mission to ensure that you see a pelvic floor physio, regardless of how or when you birthed. Below she shares some insights based on her experience as both a physio, and as a mother who has experienced pelvic organ prolapse.

There are so many ways your pelvic floor links with your entire body, your sense of self, your femininity, your intimacy and relationships. I see women as old as sixty in my clinic, only now coming to a diagnosis of pelvic floor dysfunction after decades of symptoms. Almost daily I hear 'If only someone told me' or 'If only I knew' and it breaks my heart that these women have sacrificed so many years of good health because they weren't given the care they needed and deserved.

No matter how much society has tried to normalise light bladder leakage and make it sound dainty and expected, it still is an event of urinary incontinence and not something you should be expected to just live with because you had a baby.

The steps we take for our pelvic health now set the path for our quality of life in twenty, forty, sixty years' time. Our ability to seek care and undergo pelvic rehab will help our sense of self and strength as we age, reduce our risk of falls and hospitalisation when we are elderly and play a part in being able to live at home independently for as long as we wish.

While pelvic floor dysfunction is a good indicator that you need to see a pelvic floor physio, other indicators include healing from birth injuries, returning to exercise, pain in other parts of the body, or simply for peace of mind.

Pelvic floor dysfunction might look or feel like:

- A sense of heaviness or dragging in your vagina or anus
- Pain in the pelvis, vagina or rectum
- Lower back pain
- Visible changes (some women can see their prolapse)
- Pressure in the vagina or rectum
- Vaginal farts during walking, exercise or sex – especially if they get 'stuck'
- Discomfort during sex
- Difficulty inserting tampons or menstrual cups
- Urinary incontinence or a sudden urgency to void (urge incontinence) after coughing, sneezing, laughing, lifting your baby, getting in and out of your chair (stress incontinence), or difficulty emptying your bladder and feeling you need to go again shortly after your toilet time (urinary retention)
- Constipation or faecal incontinence including involuntary opening of your bowels, a sense of urgency when you need to poo, or feeling like you can't wipe all the stool away.

Pelvic floor rehab is so much more than doing your Kegels because symptoms can be as varied as the underlying diagnosis. A session with your pelvic health physio will include things such as:

- A thorough history to gain an understanding of your life, your dreams and goals, your pregnancy, your birth, your plans for exercise, your daily tasks and movements
- An internal physical exam (with your consent)
- An ultrasound assessment
- An assessment of bladder function
- Assessment of your abdominals and core
- The opportunity to debrief about your birth
- A discussion of the findings and setting goals
- Trialling devices such as pessaries or a dilator.

Rehab will include physical strengthening or down training (pelvic floors can be overly taut or weak), learning how to monitor your symptoms, modifying daily tasks and movements, body awareness education. Ultimately, the goal is to manage pain and address your symptoms or refer you to healthcare providers when necessary. Additionally, strength or Pilates based exercises are extremely helpful in guarding against pelvic weakness, and can accelerate your postpartum recovery.

You created life, you brought that life into your arms. You are mother, you are divine feminine. You deserve to feel strong, beautiful, loved, confident and free to live your life and achieve all of your daily and motherly tasks without pain, without worrying about symptoms and feeling disconnected from your own body. You deserve to be held and helped by your pelvic health physiotherapist.

POSTPARTUM RECOVERY TIMELINE

It takes between nine and ten months to grow and birth a baby, and it therefore makes sense that the healing and recovery from pregnancy and birth will take time, dedication and compassion towards yourself as you heal and replenish.

Be gentle with yourself through this tender process. All good things take time and it is important to put your health first, with the support of your community, so that you can feel healthy, strong and vital in the months and years after the birth of your baby.

Factors that influence recovery include:

- The length and intensity of labour
- Interventions during labour and birth including epidural, forceps and vacuum
- Surgery and injury, including tears, episiotomy and caesarean
- Blood loss.

Here is an approximate timeline of what to expect from your body as it recovers in the first few weeks, months and years of the postpartum – always taking into consideration that everyone heals differently, just as they birth differently – some faster and some slower than others.

BIRTH TO 2 WEEKS

- Your uterus contracts and shrinks from the size of a watermelon to a pear. Immediately after birth you will look six months pregnant, and over the days and weeks that follow, your belly will slowly 'deflate' as your uterus returns to its pre-baby size.
- The placental wound heals and lochia discharge is at its heaviest.
- Organs are reorienting and returning to their normal place.
- Connective tissue and ligaments begin to repair and recover.
- Swelling and bruising is intense for a few days then subsides.
- Perineal grazes, tears and caesarean wounds and sutures feel tender and itchy as they heal.
- Oestrogen and progesterone levels decrease while increased prolactin stimulates breastmilk production.
- Insulin sensitivity improves after delivery of the placenta, helping to regulate blood sugar.
- The body often feels sore and you might experience joint instability due to elevated levels of relaxin.
- You may experience night sweats.
- Baby blues can occur, making you weepy and emotional.
- Hunger is high due to physical recovery and breastfeeding, which has high nutritional requirements.

Placenta Encapsulation:

Consuming the placenta after birth, something many mammal species do, has been practised in Traditional Chinese Medicine (TCM) for centuries and is becoming increasingly popular for mothers in Western society. Placenta encapsulation involves drying the placenta, grinding it into a powder and placing it in a capsule, to be consumed in the months after birth. Although extensive studies have not been undertaken into the benefits of placenta consumption, there is overflowing anecdotal evidence from mothers that it increases breastmilk, slows postpartum bleeding, boosts energy and supports mood regulation. As the placenta is an organ, it is important to ensure it is stored and handled correctly before being encapsulated to minimise risk of contamination.

THE FIRST 6 WEEKS

- Breastmilk supply establishes while mother and baby bond.
- Stitches and grazing have generally healed by the end of the first six weeks.
- Initial pelvic floor and abdominal healing is generally complete – a pelvic floor check with a health professional is recommended for assessment of diastasis, scar tissue, pelvic floor etc.
- Baby blues should lift as hormones regulate. Ongoing anxiety, depression or mood irregularities should be shared with a trusted professional.
- Lochia has generally ceased by the end of the first six weeks.
- See page 111 for a list of postpartum health assessments to ask your care provider for.

3 TO 6 MONTHS

- If still breastfeeding, nutrient requirements are high and need to be supported through quality diet and supplements.
- Hair loss and shedding may start due to decreased oestrogen and progesterone. See more info overleaf.
- Exhaustion may creep in. Many mothers are fuelled by adrenaline in the first few months after birth as they establish and juggle feeding, disturbed sleep and caring for a baby. Adrenaline now subsides and fatigue sets in – this is a good time to discuss and assess thyroid and adrenal health, iron and B12 stores and mental health.
- Movement and exercise may feel better as pelvic floor heals and nutritional stores are replenished. We recommend starting slowly and intuitively.

Hot Tip:

Antibiotics serve a purpose – to kill the bad bacteria they were created to fight – however studies show that they also kill off a large number of good, health-promoting bacteria on their path of destruction, which can cause a number of other health concerns to arise. When the intricate balance of bacteria that populate your intestines (known as the gut microbiota) is compromised, this can lead to reduced immune and gut function, impaired nutrient absorption, antibiotic resistance and other health concerns. If you were administered antibiotics at any stage during pregnancy, labour or your postpartum, we highly recommend taking a good quality probiotic to restore some of the healthy bacteria in your intestines, and speak to a health practitioner about further supporting your gut health.

- Prolactin can drop and breastmilk production ease or stop as baby eats more solids and feeds become less frequent.
- Pelvic floor has generally healed.
- Sleep remains broken due to baby's developmental leaps.
- If fatigue, hair loss or weight gain/loss continue, consider speaking to a qualified practitioner to assess thyroid and other health markers.

- Breastfeeding may have slowed or ceased.
- Weight may stabilise, however this may not happen until breastfeeding stops.
- Nutritional needs return to pre-pregnancy level, after finishing breastfeeding.

Postpartum Hair Loss:

This is a big one that we have realised most new mums know nothing about until they are standing in the shower watching their precious locks flow down the drain – but did you know that postpartum hair loss is actually a (really f*cking annoying) natural response to hormonal changes your body goes through during postpartum recovery?

Let's start with some hair basics: hair follicles go through three cycles: growth (anagen), shrinkage (catagen) and rest (telogen). The latter is when you notice that your hair is shedding, or falling out.

During pregnancy, a variety of hormones rise significantly, including thyroid, progesterone, estrogen and androgens. All of these hormones affect hair, and during pregnancy alter your body's hair growth cycle by causing hair follicles to remain in the growth phase longer than normal. This leads to a reduction in the number of hairs that are shed, which increases hair fullness (hello luscious thick pregnancy hair!).

After birth, once the placenta has been delivered, progesterone and estrogen levels dramatically reduce (which is also a major cause behind the 'baby blues'). The dramatic drop of these hormones can cause your hair cycles to shift gear – meaning that all of the thick, beautiful hair that wasn't lost during pregnancy enters a 'resting' or 'telogen' phase and you finally have a mass exodus of hair from your scalp.

Research shows that this typically starts from two to five months postpartum and continues for an average of six weeks to six months. AWESOME!

A NOTE ON BED SHARING

Bed sharing has been around since time immemorial and is still practised in many cultures today. However, bringing your baby into bed with you is not recommended by medical professionals in the West, due to its association with SIDS and the perpetuation of the 'good baby' myth. While it is still unknown exactly what causes SIDS, it is thought to be due to the baby's inability to arouse from a deep sleep, with recent studies indicating the potential for genetic factors to be involved.

When practised safely, bed sharing can have innumerable benefits for both mother and baby, such as:

- Improved regulation of an infant's body temperature and breathing due to their proximity to their mother
- Improved quality of maternal sleep
- Easier night feeds and resettling
- Improved success and length of breastfeeding.

Whether we plan to or not, most of us end up bed sharing with our babies at some point in parenthood, be it intermittently or long term and whether intentionally or in a moment of desperation. If you do bed share, we insist that you adhere to the following supported safe sleeping practices to decrease known risk factors:

- Always put your baby to sleep on their back, on a clean and firm mattress (don't place anything soft under the baby, including pillows, lamb's wool or super soft mattress toppers).
- Consider using a 'secure sleeper' device that allows you to sleep safely with your baby in your bed.
- Keep your personal bedding, sheets and pillows away from baby, especially their face, and use lightweight blankets for yourself in place of heavy quilts or doonas.
- If you are not using a secure sleeper, never swaddle your baby as this prevents them from being able to move anything that may cover their face or alert you if you are getting too close. Instead, place them in a sleeping bag that keeps their arms free.
- Remove any strangling risks, including all jewellery and teething necklaces, and tie up long hair.
- It is safest for baby to sleep on the side of a bed, away from the edge, rather than between two parents. If there is a possibility your baby might roll off the bed, consider putting your mattress on the floor.
- Never bed share with your baby and other children or pets.
- Never sleep on a sofa or armchair with your baby, even if it's just a light snooze in the daytime, as they can easily slip into a position where they get trapped in the cushions or too close to the adult's skin or clothes and can't breathe.
- Never bed share if you are a smoker, smoked during pregnancy, or are under the influence of drugs, alcohol, or medication that may make you drowsy (including sleeping tablets).

Regardless of whether they are in your bed or in their own bed, it is recommended that your baby sleeps in the same room as you for at least the first six to 12 months of their life, to reduce the risk of SIDS and Sudden Unexpected Death in Infancy.

Safe Infant Sleep by Dr James J McKenna is an excellent resource if you are curious about co-sleeping or bed sharing.

Napping as a Contact Sport

During the fourth trimester, your baby wants to be as close to you as possible. Up until now all they have known is the sound of your voice, your heart, and the gurgling sounds of your insides as you digest food and pump blood around your body. They have never known hunger, nor loneliness. By keeping them close, feeding on demand and giving them as much skin-to-skin time as possible, you are giving them a gentle transition earthside and setting them up to be confident and secure little humans. You are also encouraging a healthy and steady flow of oxytocin that helps with milk production and bonding.

Some parents feel concerned that their baby wants to sleep on them and only them during the first few weeks or months of their life, but their desire to be in contact with a warm and familiar body is innate and normal. Allowing contact naps will not create bad habits, nor will it interfere with the long-term sleep independence of your child, but it can cause you to feel trapped or touched out.

As your child gets older and becomes more independent, they will want to spend less time attached to you and more time exploring, with frequent check-ins, cuddles and reassurance that all is still okay with the world. For now though, we encourage you to use your baby's sleep time to cuddle them, rest, and allow other people to feed you and tend to household chores.

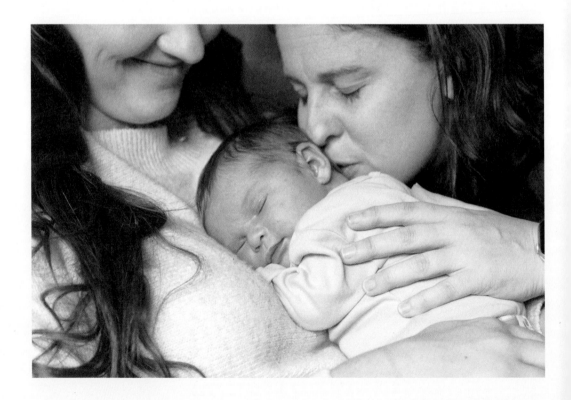

BABY WEARING

As you heal and regain strength, wearing your baby can be a great opportunity for contact naps and keeping your baby close, while also being mobile. A gentle walk, light housework or preparing a snack while wearing your baby can make a world of difference to your wellbeing and independence. Wearing your baby can also keep them out of the way of toddlers, pets and well-meaning visitors who you'd rather didn't cuddle your newborn.

While baby wearing is an excellent way of helping the mother–baby dyad to thrive, we also want to caution against the martyrdom that is entrenched in some motherhood styles. Wearing your baby all day while you walk 20,000 steps, hang out five loads of laundry, play with older children and cook a three-course meal will lead to exhaustion, back pain and possibly prolapse.

Like many things in parenthood, the reality of baby wearing can be different to how we imagined, and choosing which way you wear your baby may require trial and error until you figure out what feels best for you both. If possible, before investing in anything expensive, borrow different carriers from friends so you can see what works and what doesn't. For some, baby wearing is magic. For others, the close contact of baby and carrier can lead to sensory overwhelm, or can be plain uncomfortable. If baby wearing isn't enjoyable for both you and your baby, try a different style of carrier, or try again when they are older. You may find it helpful to visit a store where you can be taken through the different types of carriers and shown how to use them.

The three main types of baby carriers are:

- **Ergonomic baby carrier.** These have a band that goes around your hips and straps that go over your shoulders. Of all of the carriers, these are the easiest to use and the best at distributing your baby's weight evenly over your body. Many of them allow you to wear your baby facing inwards, outwards and on your back. They can be bulky, difficult to clean, and may seem way too big when your babe is still a tiny newborn, but they can be used well into the toddler years.
- **Ring sling.** This is a long piece of stiff fabric that you place over one shoulder and fasten in place with its rings. Once you figure out how to use it, a ring sling can be quick and easy to put on and adjust, but they do distribute your baby's weight unevenly and can cause back and/or hip pain when worn for extended periods of time. A bonus is that they take up very little space, and you can throw them in the washing machine with a sock over the rings.
- **Soft wrap.** These are a long piece of stretchy fabric that you wrap and tie around your body before nestling your newborn inside. They can be tricky to get the hang of, but you can tie them many ways, giving you the opportunity to change the weight distribution of your baby as often as you need. Like ring slings, they take up very little space and can be washed easily.

It can be beneficial to have different options for when you are home and when you are out, so you can mix up the ways your baby's weight is distributed across your body.

To ensure you are wearing your baby safely, remember the T.I.C.K.S. rule created by the UK Slings Consortium.

T – Carrier should be TIGHT enough to hug your baby close.
I – Baby's face should be IN view at all times.
C – Their head should be CLOSE enough to kiss.
K – KEEP baby's chin off their chest.
S – Baby's back should be SUPPORTED in its natural position with their tummy and chest against you.

HONOURING YOUR BODY

Your ripe, beautiful body has experienced and endured so much change and so much growth on the journey to becoming a mother. From the moment your baby was conceived, your body has worked tirelessly to sustain the life of another. Now that your baby is finally in your arms, your body is yours again, to navigate, to feel into, and to honour.

Many cultures around the world engage in traditional rituals and ceremonies to honour a mother and her body following the birth of her baby. These rituals bear witness to a birthing person's physical, emotional and spiritual transformation. It helps them process the birth experience and create a living memory for their baby. It provides a space for recovery, healing, reflection, acceptance and the strength to step into the next chapter.

The body is an intricate vessel that holds many stories, memories and emotions. Below are some of our favourite ways to honour your body through the postpartum; they can be undertaken at any stage, no matter when your baby was born.

Placenta Burial

In Western culture, the placenta is unfortunately considered medical waste, and is treated as such. We find this incredibly sad and astounding, given the fact that your body created its own incredible placenta to sustain your baby through pregnancy. Many cultures including Aboriginal, Torres Strait Islander, Samoan and Māori, honour this essential and sacred organ through burial ceremonies on tribal land to acknowledge the connection between mother, child, the Earth and their ancestors. Placenta burial is steeped in history and storytelling, and the process fundamentally evolves around belonging to the land and therefore finding your purpose in life. This is a beautiful alternative if you would like to keep your placenta but do not want to consume it through placenta encapsulation (see page 96).

Closing the Bones Ceremony

In Mexico la cerrada del postparto, or Closing the Bones, is a traditional midwifery practice rooted in the belief that the birthing woman's spirit undergoes great expansion to welcome the soul of the baby that has been birthed through her. It is understood that birth is a great expansion of physical, emotional and spiritual entities, and so Closing the Bones offers gentle closure to return the mother's spirit, guiding her bones, muscles and pelvic organs back into place, encouraging her uterus to shrink and promoting blood flow and warmth. The ceremony involves a ritual of blessings, candles, gentle movement, energy clearing, application of oils and massage. The mother is wrapped in traditional rebozo fabric and is honoured by wise women while she rests. Closing the Bones can also be performed to support a person after a miscarriage or abortion, and to honour the end of your breastfeeding journey or any other significant end of a cycle. In order to honour the cultural traditions of this ceremony, we recommend seeking out a practitioner who has learnt from and been given permission to facilitate Closing the Bones.

Belly Binding

The traditional practice of belly binding is an ancient art practised in Asia, Latin America and Europe, including bengkung in Malaysia and sarashi in Japan. The traditional binding technique involves using long strips of fabric which are intricately wound around a woman's abdomen for a number of health benefits. Belly binding provides gentle compression to internal organs and muscles and helps correct diastasis recti, supports posture and digestion and stabilises the nervous system by keeping the body warm. For some, using long fabric may be too labour intensive or restricting, so there are now many pre-constructed postpartum belly wraps and girdles available. Postpartum leggings also provide gentle compression.

Pelvic Steaming

Pelvic steaming has been practised throughout history by women around the world, from Central America and Eastern Europe to India and Korea. Midwives traditionally prescribed it to support healing of the vulva and reproductive organs during postpartum, as it increases warmth and circulation and may help reduce swelling, clear lochia, disinfect tears and stitches, relieve after pains and shrink haemorrhoids. Pelvic steaming often includes therapeutic herbs to offer additional nourishment plus antibacterial and lymphatic properties. After steeping the herbs in boiling water, the mother sits on a stool, chair or toilet seat over a bowl and allows the steam to deliver warmth and healing to her genital tissue and reproductive organs. The mother is wrapped in blankets or towels to seal in the heat, while sitting to pause, breathe and reflect. See recipe on page 125.

Self-massage

Birth can leave us feeling all kinds of emotions towards our bodies. For some it is a time of acceptance and coming home to self, while for others it is a time of discontent and disconnection. The practice of self-massage allows you to honour yourself and connect with your beautiful body, while offering you a daily or weekly ritual to take time for yourself and decompress. The skin is the body's largest organ, and self-massage using high-quality, organic, unrefined botanical oils promotes improved circulation while nourishing you from the outside in. Slather yourself from head to toe before or after hopping out of a warm shower to reap the beautiful benefits of this self-care practice.

Other Modalities that Support Postpartum Healing

- Acupuncture, moxibustion and cupping
- Osteopathy and craniosacral therapy
- Physiotherapy
- Chiropractic
- Massage therapy and bodywork

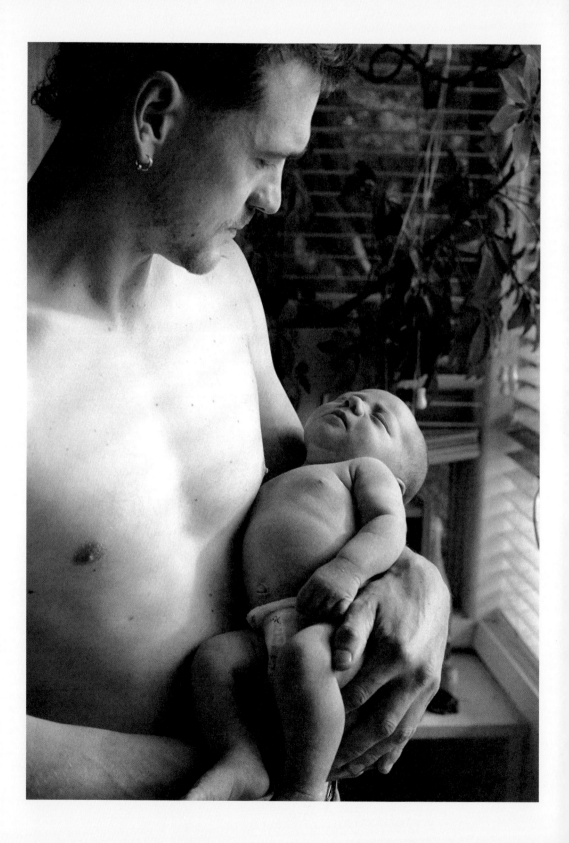

DADS AND CO-PARENTS

We cannot tell you the number of times we have had the partners of our friends and clients say to us 'I want to help, I just don't know how. I wish there was a book, or even a list in a book, that tells me what I can do to help'.

Well folks, this next section is for you.

For many, the reality of this little life that your partner has carried for the past nine months doesn't set in until you hold your baby for the first time. Most partners are utterly shook by the birth process, and after witnessing the power of the female body find themselves more in awe of and in love with their partners than ever before.

Accompanying that love and awe can be a sense of overwhelm due to the sheer responsibility of it all, and exhaustion as you come down from the emotional high and deal with your own version of sleep deprivation. Just as your partner's life has completely flipped on its head, so has yours, and you are no doubt going through a rebirth of your own.

In order for you to be the best parent and partner, you need to be resourced too. You are supporting the mother and baby, but who is supporting you? Who do you reach out to when you've had a hard day? What do you do to decompress?

At a bare minimum you need time off work to bond with your baby and support your partner, but you also need to have emotional support in place. Until now, you and your partner have had a reciprocal relationship where you care for each other's wellbeing. When your partner gave birth, this changed. They don't have the emotional and energetic reserves to care for you as well as their baby, and they probably won't for at least the first nine months but probably the first two years of your baby's life. If you have multiple children in short succession, you may find it's years before your connection and support for each other is reciprocal in the way it was before.

We also know that dads and co-parents aren't mind-readers, which is why the next section provides a framework that can help you meet your partner's needs.

The First Few Days at Home

Assuming you have a job that allows parental leave, the main role of the birthing person should be breastfeeding, eating, resting and sleeping. Everything else involved with baby care and running of the household should fall into your more-than-capable hands for now.

Things you can do to help:

- Make sure your partner is fed. There's an anecdote that says 90 per cent of arguments happen because someone is hungry. We couldn't agree more. Fellow postpartum doula Naomi Chrisoulakis shared with us the genius idea of creating a list of quick and easy to prepare nutritionally dense snacks that her partner could make for her the moment she was showing signs of 'hanger'. Everyone is different, so your partner's favourite snacks may differ to the ideas we suggest, but we share our favourites on page 231.
- Make sure your partner always has a bottle of water and/or tea, and a snack when they breastfeed. Offer to bring them their book/phone/earplugs/TV remote, and if they like to feed in a chair (as opposed to in bed) at night, get in the habit of setting up their feeding space with water, snacks, headphones and a phone charger.
- Bring them their supplements. Different supplements need to be taken at specific times of day for optimal absorption, so a hot tip is to write 'morning', 'lunch' or 'evening' on the lids in a permanent marker so it's easy for you to remember.
- Get your hands (and clothing) dirty! Burp your baby after/between feeds and take care of all nappy changes. Offer to take care of bath time too, however this may be something that mum wants to be involved with, so check first.
- Pop your baby in a carrier or take off your shirt and place them on your chest and tell mum to go and take a long shower and/or nap.
- Clean, clean, clean. Every time you leave a room, scan it for empty cups, used dishes, dirty nappies, breast pads, tissues or gift wrapping. Take out the trash, discard dead flowers, change the flower water if it's starting to get stinky and generally keep the space clutter free.
- Water the plants. There is nothing sadder than watching your beloved plants wither before your very eyes, because you are too preoccupied to water them.
- Stay on top of the laundry. Find a system that works for you and make it your thing. Managing to wash, dry, fold and put away a load of laundry (or three) in one day is a massive feat. If you can do this, we think you are f*cking superhuman and we know your partner will too.
- If you have other children, be their primary caregiver. Cover any day care and school drop offs, and on the days they aren't away, keep them entertained with trips to the playground and lots of playtime. Check in with your partner to see how much one on one time their nervous system can manage on any particular day, and help her carve out the time to make this happen by taking the newborn while she spends time with your other children.
- Whatever you do, DON'T SAY YOU'RE TIRED. You will be, but choosing to share this with other family members or friends is wise for now, as everything you are feeling is intensified a thousandfold for the person who just gave birth.

When You Go Back to Work

The prospect of being home alone with a newborn can be terrifying, especially if there are other children who need caring for as well. Ask your partner to create a list of things you can do before you leave the house to help them feel set up for the day. This may include:

- Feeding and dressing older children
- Loading/unloading the dishwasher
- Making mum breakfast or a cup of tea
- Taking out the trash
- Feeding pets
- Grabbing dinner out of the freezer
- Making sure there is something for mum to eat for lunch (hint – don't eat the dinner leftovers).

Depending on what time you start work, you may be able to help by taking the baby after their morning feed and letting mum sleep until the next feed is due or you need to go to work. Something to note – check with mum before taking baby out of the home as she could wake up and freak out. While your intentions are good, postpartum hormones can cause separation anxiety.

Last but not least, we cannot stress how important it is to keep checking in with your partner – and with yourself – to ensure that you are both on the same page and feeling supported. While you may not agree on everything, keeping the lines of communication open and trying to understand the other person's experience and perspective is vital for keeping your connection strong. If you haven't already read the first chapter of this book, we highly recommend doing so for a crash course on all things 'baby brain', relationships and personal growth.

Certain neurological changes take place during pregnancy that catalyse enormous personal growth in the gestational parent. It is normal for one partner to take the lead when it comes to personal growth while the other catches up at their own pace, but being in a different growth phase to your partner for an extended amount of time can be difficult and cause you to feel lonely and disconnected. Long-term relationships require frequent and ongoing work, both on yourself and with one another.

Hot Tip:

Make your partner a cuppa and pop it in an insulated reusable cup.

It means their drink will stay warm, and they are less likely to spill it when baby kicks or wriggles.

Genius, no?

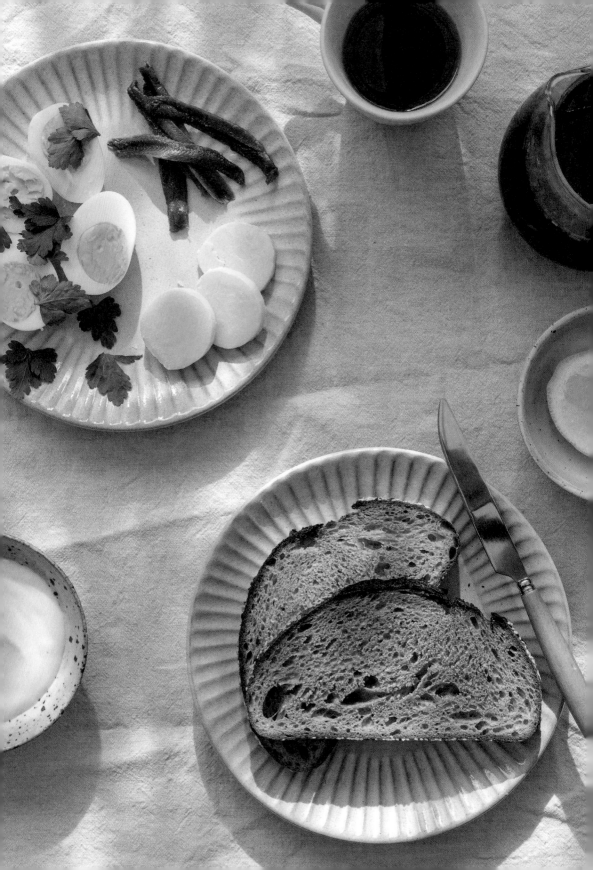

POSTPARTUM NUTRITION

CHAPTER FOUR

AND HERBAL SUPPORT

The human body is incredibly smart in its design of growing a baby. A mother provides all of the essential nutrients her baby needs via the placenta, which in turn allows the baby to develop at appropriate milestones throughout pregnancy. This is essentially a sharing or 'stealing' of nutrients from a mother's own stores, which, if not replenished through a nutrient-dense diet and supplementation both through pregnancy and the postpartum, can become increasingly low and cause health concerns, including postnatal depletion.

Postnatal depletion – a term coined by Dr Oscar Serrallach – is increasingly common in mothers and can involve symptoms of fatigue, exhaustion and the classically coined 'baby brain', which often presents with poor memory and concentration alongside emotional fragility. All of these factors have the ability to accumulate and snowball over a period of weeks, months, and even years of sleeplessness, breastfeeding, poor nutrition, subsequent hormonal imbalances and juggling the load of motherhood.

Recent studies in Australia have advised that the most heightened cases of postnatal depression appear FOUR YEARS after the birth of a child, not just the first six months, which was previously thought. This is believed to be an accumulative effect of severe postnatal depletion, which results from the way we care for ourselves (or do not) and experience care by health providers and our community during pregnancy, the birth process and the postpartum.

Most pregnancies will involve approximately twelve check-up visits with a health professional, whereas the postpartum involves several in the first week, and then often only one at six weeks, leaving new mothers without ongoing support and guidance for their wellbeing, despite now having to care not only for themselves, but their baby.

The blood tests opposite are an ideal place to start investigating any health concerns you may have, and ideally before you experience any symptoms as a way of preventative health. Your health is your wealth, so find a health practitioner that you trust and who is willing to answer all your questions, deep dive and discover anything they don't know the answer to.

In Australia, many of these can be bulk-billed by your doctor, however you may need to pay for some privately. Having a full picture of your health, especially after pregnancy and birth (and before you have another baby if this is on the cards for you) is immensely important.

POSTPARTUM HEALTH ASSESSMENTS

Blood Tests

- Vitamin D
- Full iron studies
- Full blood count
- Vitamin B12
- Thyroid panel – TSH, free T3, free T4, reverse T3, thyroid antibodies
- Liver function
- Kidney panel
- Fasting glucose
- Fasting insulin
- Plasma zinc + serum copper

Hormone Testing

Hormones generally begin to return to normal levels at approximately six months postpartum, as babies shift from exclusive breastfeeding to eating solids and maternal prolactin levels start to drop. Some mothers will experience a return of their menstrual cycle around this time, however it can come earlier or much later, and your periods may not be regular for several months as hormones rebalance themselves. Hormonal imbalance often drives symptoms such as lethargy, brain fog, difficulty concentrating, irritability, heavy and painful periods and poor libido, so if you have already had the above health markers assessed and suspect that you may have fertility or hormonal concerns, the following tests are recommended:

- Female hormones
    - Luteinising Hormones (LH)
    - Follicle Stimulating Hormone (FSH)
    - Oestradiol (taken on day 2–3 of your bleed if it has returned)
    - Progesterone (taken on day 21 of your cycle – or 7 days after you have ovulated)
- Testosterone
- Dehydroepiandrosterone (DHEAs)
- Sex Hormone Binding Globulin (SHBG)
- Prolactin
- Cortisol.

POSTPARTUM NUTRIENTS

Here is a list of some of the most essential nutrients required through the postpartum as you replenish and recover, as well as some of their food sources that you can focus on stocking in your fridge and pantry:

IRON

Iron is involved in the production of haemoglobin in red blood cells, delivering oxygen throughout your body, supporting energy production, thyroid and hormone health, as well as baby's growth and development. Blood volume increase during pregnancy, followed by blood loss during birth and breastfeeding, can all contribute to iron deficiency and anaemia. Mothers with low iron often experience symptoms including extreme fatigue, dizziness, shortness of breath and increased risk of mood disorders including depression, amongst others. Iron comes in two available sources from our diet: haem (animal products) and non-haem (plant products). Haem iron is more readily absorbed by the body, so if you follow a plant based diet, be mindful of boosting through your diet or supplementation. Combine iron rich foods with a source of vitamin C for increased absorption (think steak and broccoli), and take supplements several hours away from coffee, black tea, wine and other high tannin drinks, zinc and calcium rich foods and supplements, as these can reduce iron's absorption.

Food sources:

grass-fed red meat, liver, lentils, chickpeas, beans, tempeh, sunflower kernels, pepitas (pumpkin seeds), dried apricots, spirulina, blackstrap molasses, spinach, silverbeet (swiss chard), quinoa, tahini.

VITAMIN B12

Vitamin B12 supports the healthy production of red blood cells and initiation of tissue repair, protects your DNA from damage, as well as supports healthy immune function, energy production and cognition and nervous system regulation in both mother and baby. It is also important to have adequate levels of B12 to support the body's absorption and use of folate and iron. Vitamin B12 is obtained through the diet, primarily via animal food sources, and also created by bacteria in the gut. If you follow a plant based diet or have any digestive issues, this may require assessment and supplementation.

Food sources:

shellfish (clams, mussels, oysters, scallops), fish (salmon, Atlantic mackerel, sardines, trout, snapper), grass-fed beef, liver, eggs, cheese, nutritional yeast.

VITAMIN D

Vitamin D most famously helps to keep bones healthy and strong, but it also plays a crucial role in the body's absorption and use of calcium, iron, magnesium and zinc. What many don't know is that vitamin D is actually a hormone. It supports immune function and reduces inflammation in the body, meaning adequate stores can reduce inflammatory health concerns, including depression and auto-immune concerns that arise for mothers during their postpartum. Deficiency is common due to modern living arrangements which see many of us working and socialising indoors. Just 10–20 minutes of sun exposure each day (outside of intense UV ray times) on your exposed belly and thighs (without sunscreen) has been found to offer the best form of vitamin D repletion.

Food sources:

sardines, salmon, prawns, egg yolk, mushrooms, fortified plant based foods (e.g. grains, cereals, plant milks – be mindful of other additives such as oils and sugar).

CALCIUM

Calcium is a crucial nutrient during pregnancy and breastfeeding, as your body will quite literally draw calcium out of your bones to supply your growing baby, who will utilise it for their own bone and cardiovascular development. Ensuring you are consuming sufficient calcium will not only support your own bone density, but will promote blood clotting, muscle contraction, nervous system regulation and cardiovascular health.

Food sources:

grass-fed milk and cheese, eggs, dark leafy greens (bok choy, kale, silverbeet/swiss chard etc.), sardines, almonds, brazil nuts, beans, peas, lentils, tempeh, chia seeds, linseeds (flax seeds), sesame seeds.

MAGNESIUM

Magnesium is used and required in abundance by all bodies to support nerve function, energy production, blood sugar stability, muscle and bone health, improve 'relaxation' and 'feel-good' brain chemical production and increase melatonin production which aids sleep quality. Stress is a major cause of magnesium depletion. Low levels can cause fatigue, poor memory, concentration and mood, a hazy 'mum brain', tight and aching muscles and light, broken sleep patterns. Magnesium is best taken in glycinate and citrate form as a supplement, which are more readily absorbed and gentle on digestion.

Food sources:

nuts and seeds, whole grains, dark leafy greens, raw cacao, organic soy (tofu, tempeh, edamame), potato, brown rice, oats, banana, salmon.

FAT SOLUBLE VITAMINS: A, E, K

Vitamin A is an important nutrient for the development of breasts through all life stages, especially the physical changes that occur during breastfeeding to facilitate milk production and during the shape shifting that occurs during weaning.

Vitamin E is a potent antioxidant that supports the health of cell membranes and is found abundantly in colostrum, therefore adequate maternal stores are required.

Vitamin K2 is essential to support the delivery and uptake of calcium into bones and teeth of both mother and baby, as well as for healthy blood clotting.

Vit A food sources:

organ meat, chicken, grass-fed beef, free-range egg yolk, aged cheese, fermented foods including natto (fermented soybeans).

Vit E food sources:

sunflower kernels, almonds, hazelnuts, pine nuts, peanuts, abalone.

Vit K2 food sources:

leafy greens, natto, organic liver, prunes, kiwifruit, cheese.

TRACE MINERALS: IODINE, SELENIUM

Trace minerals, including iodine and selenium, are required in small and specific amounts, yet do very important and specific jobs within the organs and systems of the body.

Iodine is required for healthy hormone production, especially the thyroid which regulates our metabolism and energy. It is also vital for immune function, alongside breast and ovarian health.

Selenium plays a significant role in reducing inflammation and has been found to support auto-immune and thyroid conditions, alongside postpartum depression. It is also useful for regulating cholesterol and protecting against heavy metal exposure.

Iodine food sources:

seaweed (kelp, nori, kombu, wakame), fish and shellfish, eggs, liver.

Selenium food sources:

brazil nuts, cottage cheese, eggs, brown rice, sunflower kernels, poultry, grass-fed beef, pork.

OMEGA 3 ESSENTIAL FATTY ACIDS (EFAs)

Omega 3 EFAs, specifically DHA (docosahexaenoic acid) are required and used abundantly throughout pregnancy and the postpartum by babies for the healthy development of the nervous system, brain and eyes, and by mothers to protect neurons in the brain for healthy mental functioning and mood regulation, as well as postpartum oestrogen production. A deficiency of EFAs can contribute to classic symptoms of 'baby brain' including reduced mental clarity, poor memory and fogginess, as well as mood disorders including anxiety and hormonal imbalances. The human body cannot synthesise EFAs and they must therefore be consumed as part of a healthy diet or through supplementation to ensure that both mother and baby receive optimal levels.

Food sources:

mackerel, salmon, sardines, anchovies, trout, cod liver oil, linseeds (flax seeds), chia seeds, hemp seeds, walnuts and algae.

VITAMIN C

Vitamin C supports the maintenance of elasticity and collagen production within the skin and ligaments of the body, which is particularly important in the postpartum. Vitamin C also supports energy production and acts to support the adrenal glands. High concentrations are required by the brain for the production of mood enhancing and calming neurotransmitters, including serotonin, melatonin and dopamine. Additionally, it is a potent antioxidant that protects the body from inflammation and supports immune function, while aiding the absorption of iron.

Food sources:

citrus fruits, kiwi fruit, capsicum (bell peppers), strawberries, papaya, tomatoes, cruciferous vegetables (broccoli, kale, cauliflower etc.), kakadu plum, rosehips.

ZINC

Zinc is involved in maintaining a robust immune system, helps create DNA and chemical messengers that regulate mood, and supports hormone and digestive health. Zinc can be difficult for the gut to absorb so, much like iron, it requires a healthy amount of stomach acid to be properly utilised. It is important to note that low levels of zinc can allow for one of its major competitors – copper – to become present in high levels, which has been found to increase the risk of postpartum depression, obsessive and compulsive thoughts, inflammation and hormonal imbalances.

Food sources:

oysters, crab, lobster, poultry, beef, pork, eggs, pepitas (pumpkin seeds), pine nuts, lentils and beans, oats, chia seeds, quinoa, shiitake mushrooms, spinach.

B VITAMINS

B Vitamins are essential building blocks of energy production and mood, including the healthy function of neurotransmitters, including serotonin which regulates feelings of happiness and reduces feelings of stress and depression. Specific B vitamins also work to regulate blood sugar, cortisol and adrenal gland health, magnesium levels in the body and the way we process carbohydrates. Some people are genetically predisposed to difficulty processing certain B vitamins (specifically B9 or 'folate'), so it is recommended to take an activated form of B vitamin supplements.

Food sources:

leafy greens, green peas, avocado, nutritional yeast, brown rice, eggs, natural yoghurt, legumes, mussels, clams, oysters, salmon, trout, beef, poultry.

CHOLINE

Choline is essential during pregnancy and the postpartum for continuous infant memory and brain development, gene expression and DNA formation amongst others. It has been found in abundance in breastmilk, and therefore maternal requirements, especially during lactation, are exceptionally high and need to be replenished through the diet and supplementation to provide a growing baby the building blocks it needs for physical and cognitive growth.

Food sources:

egg yolk, liver, beef, chicken, salmon, legumes, cruciferous vegetables, sunflower lecithin.

PLANT MEDICINE FOR MOTHERHOOD

In many cultures throughout history, women and especially mothers have gathered plants and prepared herbal medicine as a way of tending to their bodies, babies and community. What is nowadays deemed as alternative medicine is in fact utilising the knowledge our ancestors had of our symbiotic relationship with the environment. Thanks to our rich knowledge of plants, combined with the ingenuity of modern science, there is an abundance of growing evidence on the biological and physiological ways herbal medicine can support reproductive health. This is the basis on which Vaughne practises naturopathy, and she has seen SO many women and mothers benefit from the therapeutic use of plant medicine.

Mother Nature truly does appear in all her glory during the reproductive phases of a woman's life. Despite the modernity that surrounds us and the busy, technology-driven lives we lead, our bodies still function to the cyclical ebb and flow of nature. To this day, just as they always have, human babies are carried in the womb for approximately ten moon phases and during that time a mother's biology innately grows and nourishes the foetus using her nutritional stores.

It is easy to lose sight of just how natural the process of childbearing and birthing is. However you birth your baby, whether vaginally or via caesarean, the innate process of growing your baby and producing milk is an extraordinary feat of nature.

Connecting with the Earth, which sustains the human race, seems to become more apparent and important to mothers after the birth of their child. The cyclical process of preparing for and planting your own seeds (egg and sperm) for a successful conception, tending to yourself and your baby with the tools you have during pregnancy (nutrition, supplements, exercise, bodywork, emotional support) and watching your belly grow and bloom as weeks roll into months all unfold as if by magic. But it also evokes an ancient and wise element within mothers that connects them to one another, their own feminine lineage, and to an appreciation for elements of nature that offer grounding, nourishment, healing and respite during a time of great upheaval and transformation.

Using herbal medicine as part of your postpartum care is a gentle and environmentally conscious approach that connects you with nature. Herbs and plant medicine in the form of teas, tinctures and topical treatments offer an incredible variety of therapeutic benefits. They contain vitamins, minerals and restorative properties that have a profoundly positive effect on female reproductive health, and science is continuously recognising that they support a multitude of postpartum health concerns and the general wellbeing of mother and baby.

While we are deeply grateful for and pay great reverence to modern medicine, herbal medicine is complimentary, preventative and can be easily incorporated into your everyday life. Following the physical and emotional changes that take place during birth and in early postpartum, we wholeheartedly believe in going back to basics and minimising exposure of chemicals for you and your sensitive baby. Using the wisdom of nature to support your healing is a powerful way to encourage hormones, your nervous system and your body as a whole to recalibrate as you embrace motherhood.

Postpartum Herbal Apothecary

Creating your own herbal remedies is incredibly easy and satisfying, especially when using the simple yet effective therapeutic properties of dried herbs. Liquid herbal tinctures contain potent and intricate botanical medicinal properties that should be prescribed by a qualified naturopath or herbalist, however dried herbs are a readily accessible option for anyone at home and can become star players in your medicine cabinet that you feel confident using on a regular basis.

Dried herbs have a long shelf life and can be sourced from your local health food store or a variety of online dispensaries. Organic varieties are best, as they are grown using the least amount of chemicals and pesticides, and are best stored in glass jars, out of direct sunlight.

Below are some of our favourite herbs that are easily accessible in most pockets of the world. Use these to create teas and topical treatments to soothe, restore, repair and replenish when the mood or ailment strikes.

- Alfalfa
- Calendula
- Chamomile
- Echinacea
- Fennel
- Fenugreek
- Ginger
- Lavender
- Lemon balm
- Motherwort
- Nettle
- Oat straw
- Raspberry leaf
- Rose
- Rosemary
- Skullcap
- Thyme
- Vervain
- Witch-hazel
- Yarrow

Although this list is not exhaustive, some herbs may be dangerous when transferred to babies via breastmilk, so consult with a qualified herbalist before consuming teas or tinctures containing the following:

- Aloe
- Bearberry
- Black cohosh
- Bladderwrack
- Buckthorn
- Comfrey
- Dong quai
- Elecampane
- Ginseng
  (Siberian is OK)
- Goldenseal
- Kava
- Prickly ash
- Rhubarb
- Senna
- Tobacco
- Wintergreen
- Wormwood

Essential Postpartum Supplements & Remedies

Here, we've put together a list of our favourite remedies that we recommend to our doula clients time and time again through the postpartum to support basic recovery.

We acknowledge that no two mothers will experience the same physical and emotional symptoms during their postpartum. In order to receive the individualised health care that you so greatly deserve, we recommend seeking support from a qualified practitioner. In cases where this isn't financially possible, look for a health food store that sells practitioner-only supplements – they will usually have a naturopath working on the floor who can offer you personalised recommendations.

In order to receive the highest quality supplements possible, we recommend avoiding generic supermarket or chemist brands, as these often contain inadequate amounts and poorly absorbed forms of vitamins, minerals and antioxidants that are required by you and your baby.

- **Magnesium** – this wonderful nutrient supports the nervous system, energy production and muscular aches during the postpartum. Magnesium glycinate is a well absorbed and tolerated supplement form.
- **Arnica** – this homeopathic remedy is used to reduce bruising and swelling of the perineum and other tissues after birth. It can be taken as drops or in pill form.
- **Vitamin C** – is an important nutrient and antioxidant required for tissue repair and wound healing, collagen synthesis and immune support, while helping to increase the absorption of iron.
- **Probiotics** – a quality probiotic supplement containing Lactobacillus and Bifidobacterium strains support gut flora balance. Studies show that consuming probiotics has a multitude of benefits for both mother and baby, including improved digestive and immune health.
- **Breastfeeding-friendly multivitamin** – we recommend continuing to take your pregnancy multivitamin while breastfeeding, as they contain a variety of essential nutrients that your body requires in abundance during this time.
- **Echinacea tincture and tea** – this herb contains active properties that support immune health and help fight infection. It is safe to take while breastfeeding and is a wonderful ally during bouts of mastitis or when you are feeling run down.

Medicinal Cannabis

Although there is still societal stigma surrounding cannabis, this medicinal plant has long been used as part of women's health to relieve menstrual cramps, anxiety, insomnia, chronic pain and nausea, amongst other ailments and conditions. With more and more studies supporting its therapeutic use, Cannabidiol (CBD) and Tetrahydrocannabinol (THC) are increasingly being prescribed by medical practitioners.

While some medical cannabis contains THC – the psychoactive compound that makes you high – you can also consume it in CBD form, which has all of the therapeutic benefits, but none of the psychoactive properties.

If you suffer from any of the conditions listed above, you may wish to look into medicinal cannabis as a tool for managing your symptoms.

'I cannot stress strongly enough how positive cannabis has been for my motherhood journey. It is not about zoning out or escaping, quite the opposite! On days where my kids are doing my head in with their constant bickering and intense demands, cannabis allows me to calm down, drop in, and be a more present and intuitive mother.' – Jess

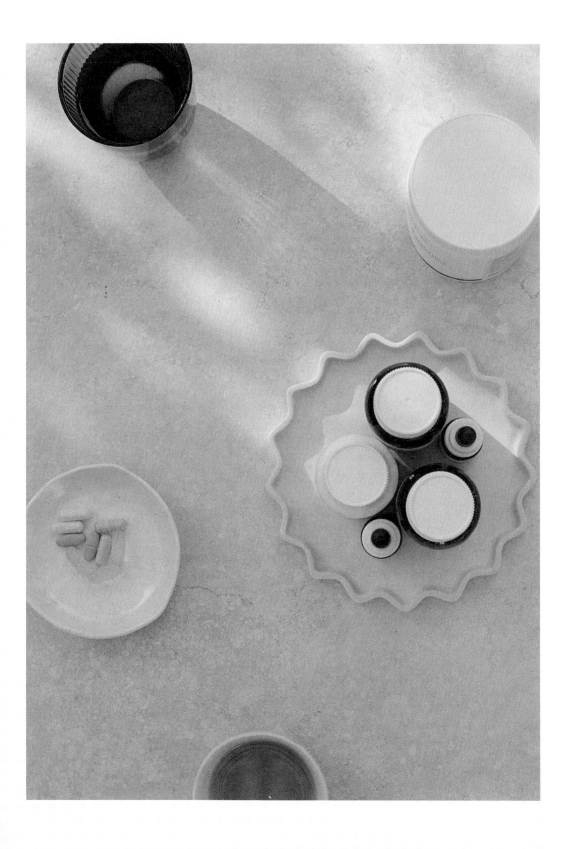

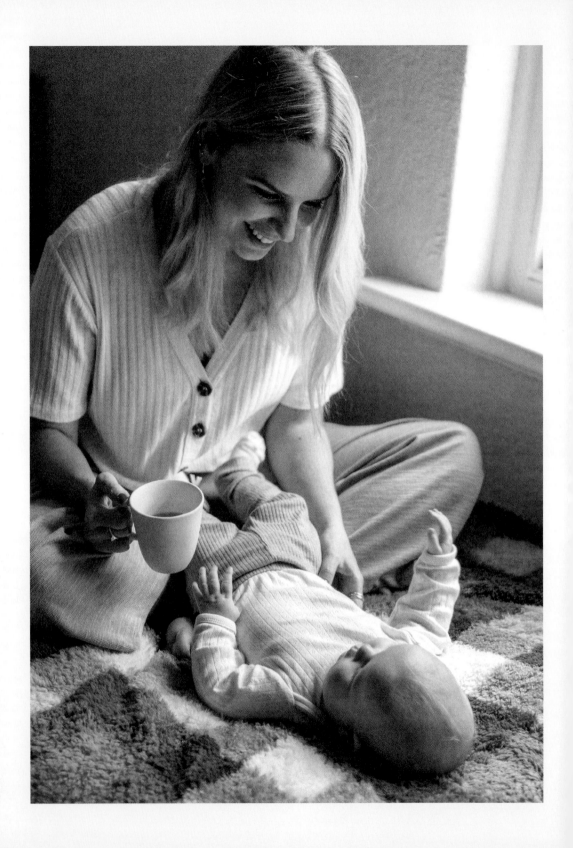

TEA, GLORIOUS TEA

Below are some of our favourite herbal recipes that we recommend preparing during pregnancy, so you can call on the therapeutic and hydrating power of tea during the postpartum. For each recipe, combine herbs in a bowl and store in an airtight glass jar.

Afterbirth Tea

3 tablespoons dried raspberry leaf
3 tablespoons dried motherwort
3 tablespoons dried chamomile
3 tablespoons dried nettle
2 tablespoons dried ginger

Breastfeeding Tea

3 tablespoons fennel seeds
2 tablespoons fenugreek seeds
3 tablespoons dried alfalfa
3 tablespoons dried vervain
3 tablespoons dried nettle

Calming Tea

3 tablespoons dried lemon balm
3 tablespoons dried oat straw
3 tablespoons dried rose
3 tablespoons dried chamomile
3 tablespoons dried vervain

Digestive Tea

3 tablespoons dried chamomile
3 tablespoons dried lemon balm
3 tablespoons fennel seeds
2 tablespoons dried ginger
3 tablespoons dried vervain

Mastitis Tea

3 tablespoons dried echinacea
3 tablespoons dried thyme
3 tablespoons dried lemon balm
2 tablespoons dried rosemary
2 tablespoons dried ginger

MAKES 1 CUP

1 tablespoon herbal tea
1 cup water, boiled

Place the tea in a teapot or strainer and cover with the water.

Steep for 5 to 10 minutes then pour through a strainer to separate the herbs from the liquid.

Enjoy hot, warm or cold.

Drink 2 to 4 cups daily.

Tips:

- You will need 1 tablespoon of loose tea per cup of hot water.
- The longer you infuse the herbs, the stronger the brew, both in flavour and medicinal strength.
- Add a squeeze of lemon or honey for taste. We love active manuka honey, which contains anti-inflammatory, antibacterial and immune supporting properties.

HERBAL PERI PADS

Herbal Peri Pads are renowned for their ability to cool and soothe the tender perineum that many people experience following a vaginal birth. You may feel a bit bruised and swollen in the week after birth and these are the perfect way to bring some comfort using natural ingredients that won't irritate the delicate skin and tissue. This recipe calls for dried witch-hazel. You can also use witch-hazel distillate, just make sure it's an alcohol free one (because, ouch!).

3 tablespoons dried lavender
3 tablespoons dried calendula flowers
3 tablespoons dried chamomile
3 tablespoons dried witch-hazel
1 packet maternity pads
pure aloe vera gel

Make your herbal infusion by placing dried lavender, calendula, chamomile and witch-hazel in a heat-proof vessel and cover with 1 litre (34 fl oz/4 cups) of boiled water. Stir well, cover, and allow to steep for 20 minutes.

Strain the herbal infusion into a measuring jug or glass jar and leave on the bench to cool. Discard the herbs in your compost or garden.

Unfold each pad, leaving them attached to the wrapping.

Pour approximately 2 tablespoons of herbal infusion evenly across each pad, ensuring they are damp but not saturated as you want to leave some absorbency for postpartum bleeding.

Using a knife, spread a thin layer of aloe vera gel on each pad to cover the surface.

Rewrap the pads loosely in their wrapper and pop them in a container in the freezer for at least 4 hours to cool.

To use, place the pad as you would normally in your underwear (or adult diapers which are amazing in the first week after birth to prevent leaking).

Save any remaining herbal liquid in a jar and pop in the fridge. This can be used in a peri bottle, for more peri pads, or added to a warm bath with magnesium flakes for a soothing herbal soak.

Note:
Peri pads should be used to offer soothing relief, but be mindful to remove them once they are no longer cool as your vagina and perineum should not be exposed to moisture for long periods of time while healing, as it can increase risk of infection.

HERBAL SITZ

If you have experienced grazing, tearing, tenderness, swelling or haemorrhoids (who hasn't!) following birth, a herbal sitz is your best friend. The warmth of the water brings blood flow while these herbs are soothing, calming, astringent, antibacterial and healing to all your tender bits. We have written this recipe for use in a bath, however you can also purchase a sitz-bath accessory for your toilet, which allows your genitals to submerge in warm water. This recipe can also be used in a peri bottle.

3 tablespoons dried calendula
3 tablespoons dried chamomile
3 tablespoons dried lavender
3 tablespoons dried rosemary
3 tablespoons dried witch-hazel
3 tablespoons dried yarrow
400 g (14 oz/2 cups) Epsom salts (magnesium sulfate)

Add the dried herbs to a large pot or glass bowl, add 500 ml (17 fl oz/2 cups) boiling water, stir well, cover, and allow to steep for 20 minutes.

Using a tea strainer or fine-mesh sieve, strain the herbal infusion into a measuring jug or glass jar and allow to cool. Discard the herbs in your compost or garden.

Run a shallow, warm bath approximately 5 cm (2 in) high. Add the Epsom salts and swirl the water until dissolved.

Pour the herbal infusion into the magnesium bath and sit for 10 to 15 minutes. Repeat daily to support healing.

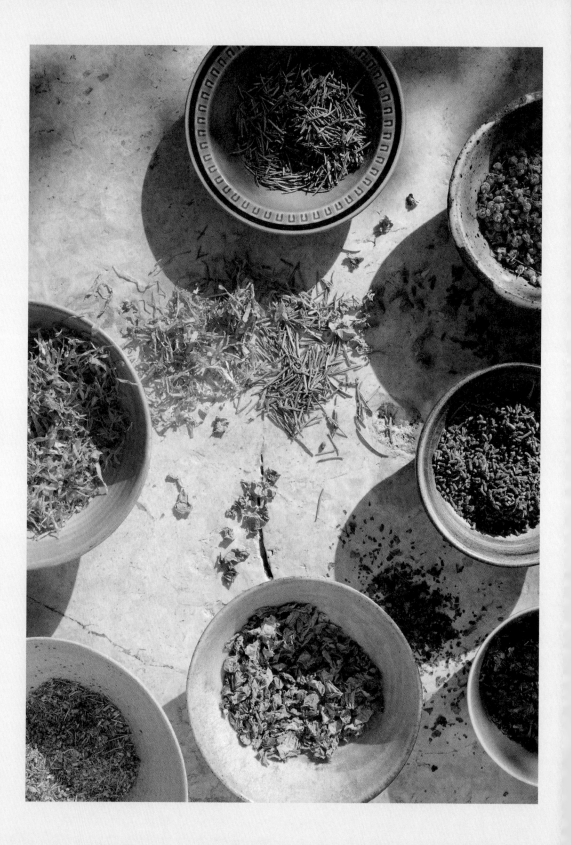

HERBAL PELVIC STEAM

Pelvic steaming may seem a bit *new-age-woo-woo* but it's rooted in history and has been used by midwives since well before they were being burnt at the stake. Pelvic steaming delivers therapeutic warmth to the vulva, anus and delicate tissue of the reproductive organs, and the addition of herbs provides circulatory, lymphatic, anti-microbial and nourishing properties. It is recommended to wait until your lochia has started to ease before steaming, generally by the end of the first 7–10 days after birth, as this means that your uterine artery has started to close. It is important to speak with your midwife or health professional about when is safe for you to start, as it may differ from mother to mother based on your birth experience, recovery and any injuries.

1 litre (34 fl oz/4 cups) water
3 tablespoons dried lavender
3 tablespoons dried motherwort
3 tablespoons dried raspberry leaf
3 tablespoons dried rose
3 tablespoons dried rosemary
3 tablespoons dried thyme

In a medium pot, bring the water to a boil and reduce to a simmer. Add herbs, stir, cover, and allow to simmer for 10 minutes. Remove from the heat and allow to steep for a further 10 minutes.

Pour the herbal liquid into a stainless steel mixing bowl and using your wrist, check the temperature of the steam to make sure it is not too hot and feels comfortable enough to sit over.

Place the bowl under a steaming stool (with a hole in it) or alternatively use your toilet, ensuring the toilet is sanitised. Place the stainless steel bowl in the toilet bowl (put the toilet lid up before doing this) so that it is sitting above the water and steam is rising. Lower the toilet seat and sit on the toilet. Wrap your upper body and legs in a warm blanket or towel and sit over the steam for 10 to 15 minutes.

Caution:
- *Do not sit directly over hot steam – it should feel warm and comfortable.*
- *Do not use essential oils as they are too harsh for the delicate tissue of the reproductive tissue and organs. Use the 'whole herb principle' and stick with dried herbs.*
- *Do not steam if you have any internal or external infection.*

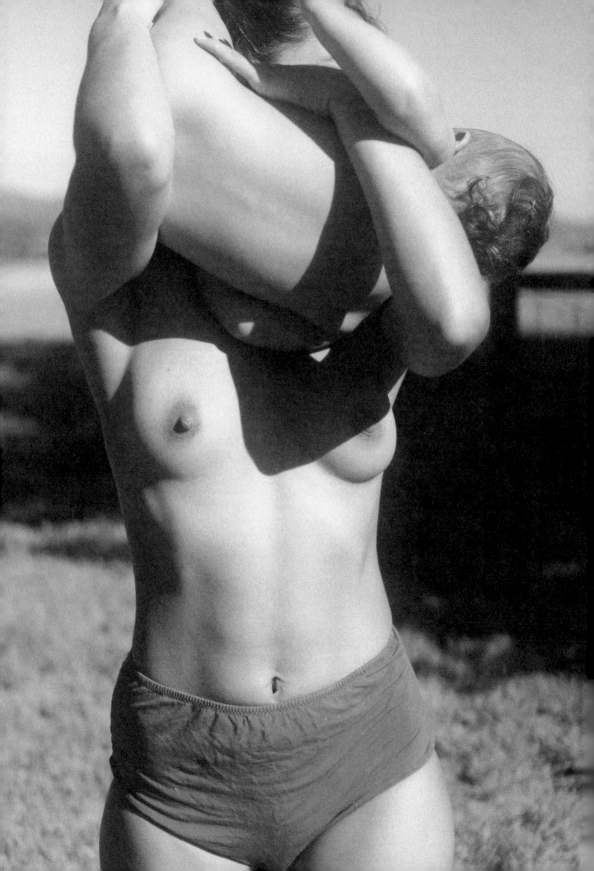

POSTPARTUM

CHAPTER FIVE

IS FOREVER

There is a strange societal expectation that once you've had your six-week check-up, you're supposed to slide into your jeans and glide into your favourite cafe with your baby sleeping peacefully in their pram.

For most, this could not be further from the truth. And yet, the narrative remains that to achieve all this makes you a super mum, a superhuman, a warrior. This narrative is deeply detrimental to the wellbeing of our culture. If you haven't heard us drumming it into you yet, new mums and birthing people need rest and, contrary to what the media portrays, most new parents are still fumbling their way through life well beyond the first six weeks. Switching to a slower, more child-led rhythm may come as a shock to many, who find that all of a sudden, getting out of the house with a newborn is a full-time job, and making food when you have a clingy baby is next to impossible.

This chapter is about how to step out of your fourth trimester and into your forever postpartum as a wiser and stronger version of yourself. In these pages we share tips on how to survive when the help falls away, your partner returns to work, your midwife and doula visits finish and the meal train stops. We also share how to survive years down the track, when you realise that the cumulative effects of broken sleep and not nourishing yourself properly have almost broken you and wrought havoc on your relationships, and that becoming a parent has completely shifted your identity.

'Because the truth is this – the first few years of postpartum are going to pull you so far away from who you used to be – and then they're going to put you back together as the person you're meant to become.'

JANUARY HARSHE, AUTHOR OF *BIRTH WITHOUT FEAR: THE JUDGMENT-FREE GUIDE TO TAKING CHARGE OF YOUR PREGNANCY, BIRTH, AND POSTPARTUM*

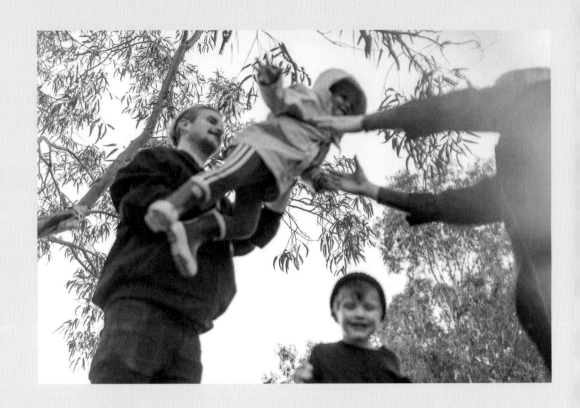

'The wellbeing of mothers is the
fabric from which the cloth of
the future of our society is made.'

DR OSCAR SERRALACH

YOUR NEW SELF

In a society where we are force-fed unrealistic body expectations, it can be difficult to know what a real body will look like after giving birth. We are bombarded with images of thin women every time we open Instagram or turn on a television, and most of us carry remnants of the glossy magazines we grew up with, all of which glorified thin. Heck, most of the world still glorifies thin, despite a strong movement encouraging women to take up space and be comfortable no matter their size. There is an inordinate amount of internal (self) and external (societal) pressure, and projected beliefs from generations before us to 'bounce back' however, we are here to challenge bounce-back culture and remind you that you should instead be bouncing forward.

In our most vulnerable moments, it's difficult not to focus on things the patriarchy tells us are negative, including weight gain, stretch marks, hair loss, leaking and lopsided boobs, hormonal skin changes and the myriad of other bodily changes we must contend with alongside the blur of sleepless nights and the shattering of our entire identity.

Some women experience only minor changes that they find liberating. They realise how freaking incredible their bodies are and enjoy being softer and feel more comfortable in their skin than ever before. For others, dare we say most, the changes that come with motherhood can be a source of anxiety, shame and can induce a lack of self-worth. Many feel defined by their weight loss or lack thereof, which can be all-consuming for those who – in a time of great unknown and change – focus on their weight as a means of feeling in control.

Start to tune into your self-talk; how do you speak to the person you see in the mirror? If they are not words you would say to a cherished friend, you should not be saying them to yourself either. Not internally, and especially not in front of your children. If we are going to break the generational cycle of diet culture and body shaming, it needs to start with us.

We've said it before but we will say it again (and again!), bounce-back culture is misguided. You are beautiful and worthy no matter how you look.

Calorie restriction, over-exercising and depriving yourself of essential food and nutrients can have detrimental effects on so many processes of motherhood. Breastmilk supply, mental health and postnatal repletion are all compromised when new mothers shift their focus from healing and bonding with their baby to fitting into those stupid pre-pregnancy jeans. You might get there one day, but the immediate postpartum is a time to celebrate your beautiful body and everything it has done for you and your baby.

Our biggest tip for managing your body image is exercise. Not because it helps regulate weight (although it can), but because most people *feel* great after they have moved their body. In a study comparing exercise with the use of antidepressants and a placebo pill, exercise was as effective as the medication. Exercise releases neurotransmitters, including endorphins, dopamine and serotonin, which combine to reduce feelings of pain and stress. It also boosts mood, while simultaneously dialling down the number of f*cks you give about the way you look. It's magic!

Studies have also shown that exercise improves sleep quality, and, importantly, it provides us with a sense of achievement. When you combine all those benefits, you can see why we think mothers (and partners) have so much to gain from moving their bodies.

Gentle reminder: it is important to make sure your pelvic floor is intact before restarting any kind of exercise, regardless of whether it's high or low intensity, so as to not cause any further issues. Speak to a trusted health professional for an assessment if you have any concerns. It's also worth noting that relaxin production continues while you are breastfeeding, so you may experience joint instability and be more susceptible to injury until you have stopped.

How to Dress Your New Body

There is a reason why leggings and sneakers are so popular with mums. They are freaking comfortable and there is a joy and efficiency that comes from a lack of restriction caused by your clothing. They are also super easy to wash, and when your child starts solids and becomes mobile, you will understand why this is helpful. But it's also important to have a couple of outfits on rotation that flatter your body and make you feel really good. We are all about the 'capsule wardrobe' which means buying less but better quality clothing. Jess calls this the uniform: choosing a select few items and unapologetically wearing them to death. You may go up a dress size or two after having a baby and this may or may not last forever. Now more than ever, it's important to remember that you are so much more than the number on an item of clothing.

'After having both my children, none of my clothing fit me. I felt frumpy and dumpy and either tragically uncool, or completely invisible to those around me. It took some time to find my groove, but I now love my body more than ever – stretch marks, saggy parts and all. What women do every day is nothing short of a miracle, and yet we are distracted from the magic of our creative power by unrealistic body standards that serve no one except the industries that profit from them.

By saying no to bounce-back culture and leaning into the new version of yourself that is stronger, wiser and softer, you are rewriting the trajectory of womanhood.

ALL bodies are beautiful, ALL bodies are worthy and ALL bodies are F*CKING INCREDIBLE.' – Jess

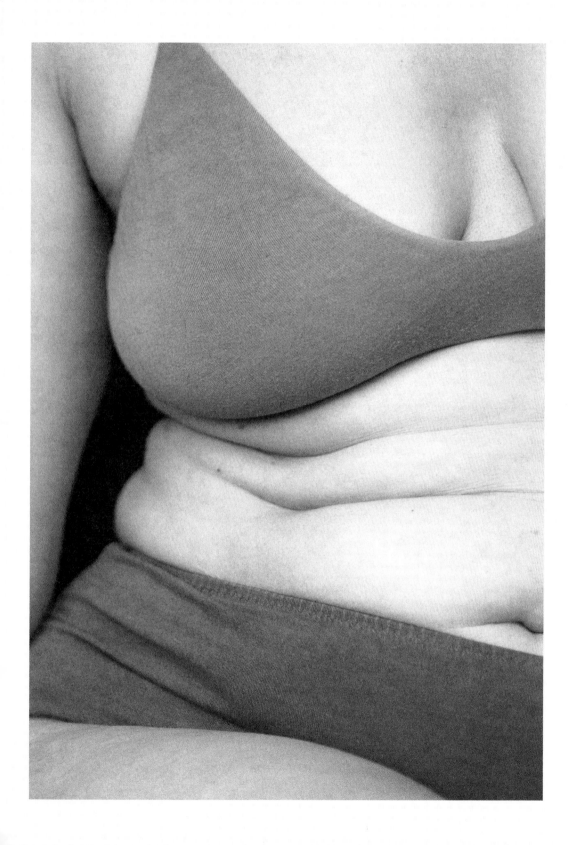

PARENTING ON YOUR PERIOD

If you are breastfeeding, it's likely your period won't return until somewhere between 6–18 months postpartum. When it does, it might be irregular and feel rather different to your pre-baby periods. Many women have heavier periods following pregnancy, as the uterus – despite how miraculously it returns to its pre-baby size – is often stretched, creating more surface area and therefore more blood as the lining of your uterus sheds. It can also be unpleasant for those who have to mitigate cramps as well as breastfeed, and even for those who get sensitive nipples when they are ovulating.

If you don't already know the concept of treating each phase of your cycle like a season, motherhood is the time to do so. The entire world exists on a linear timeline, with focus solely on the circadian rhythm of day and night. While the circadian rhythm is important, there is another rhythm that dictates the emotional, energetic and nutritional needs of people who bleed, and it's called the infradian rhythm. To some, the daily changes in energy and mood can feel manic, but when we start to pay attention to the fluctuations in our hormones, we create a deeper understanding of WHY we feel this way, which brings an ease and flow to parenthood.

Male hormonal patterns are predictable and linear; testosterone is highest in the morning and decreases in the evening. This repeats on a daily basis and has shaped the way our society operates. Women on the other hand have an intricate, cyclical pattern of hormonal interplay that ebbs and flows throughout the month. During this, oestrogen rises and falls, as do progesterone and other important fertility hormones which optimise our chances of conception. If an egg is not fertilised, they facilitate a menstrual bleed, before starting all over again. When you understand this, it is illogical that society is expected to operate on a timeline that at best only serves half the population: men.

By knowing where you are in your cycle, you can keep track of when you will have energy and when you will need rest, then plan your life accordingly. Overleaf we share what to expect from each phase of your cycle and how to harness its benefits, but we wanted to take a moment to emphasise the importance of treating the first days of your bleed like a mini-postpartum, if you may. Repeat after us: when you are bleeding it is time for deep rest. Parent from the couch, whether it be movie marathons, horizontal games, or both. Order takeout or eat those meals you filled your freezer with earlier in the month. Let the house get messy and say no to social engagements. Give yourself permission to *relax*.

'Knowing where I am in my cycle has brought an ease to parenting, as it helps me to understand why parenting is sometimes effortless and at other times it breaks me. It's helped me to know when I will enjoy socialising and when I need solitude; when to deep clean the house and fill my freezer, and when to parent from the couch and order takeout. My boys call my period my "mama blood" and are endlessly fascinated by its existence.' – Jess

---

Discussing Periods with Children:

It's important to note that children are not born with inherent shame about periods – this is something they learn from us. If you grew up in a home where periods were shameful, taboo, or simply ignored, you may be unsure how to talk about them with your own kids. Our advice: be very matter of fact about it, and if they say 'eww' or 'gross' remind them how important periods are, as they are part of the cycle that is responsible for their existence on Earth.

'The menstrual cycle is a cycle to base your life around, in fact your life is based around your menstrual cycle whether you realise it or not, whether you pay attention to it or not. And everyone who lives under the same roof is under the influence of the menstrual cycles of the women who live there. If you don't believe that, just ask them!'

JANE HARDWICKE COLLINGS, *BLOOD RITES – THE SPIRITUAL PRACTICE OF MENSTRUATION*

Phases of the Cycle

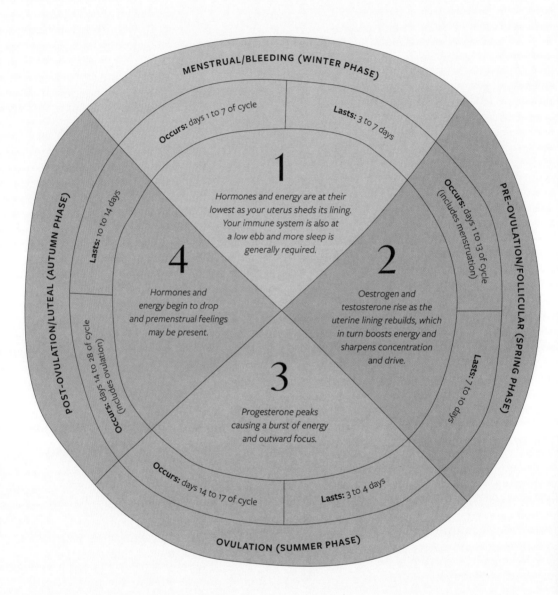

MENSTRUAL/BLEEDING (WINTER PHASE)

Occurs: days 1 to 7 of cycle

Lasts: 3 to 7 days

1

Hormones and energy are at their lowest as your uterus sheds its lining. Your immune system is also at a low ebb and more sleep is generally required.

PRE-OVULATION/FOLLICULAR (SPRING PHASE)

Occurs: days 1 to 13 of cycle (includes menstruation)

Lasts: 7 to 10 days

2

Oestrogen and testosterone rise as the uterine lining rebuilds, which in turn boosts energy and sharpens concentration and drive.

POST-OVULATION/LUTEAL (AUTUMN PHASE)

Lasts: 10 to 14 days

Occurs: days 14 to 28 of cycle (includes ovulation)

4

Hormones and energy begin to drop and premenstrual feelings may be present.

3

Progesterone peaks causing a burst of energy and outward focus.

Occurs: days 14 to 17 of cycle

Lasts: 3 to 4 days

OVULATION (SUMMER PHASE)

this is based on a regular 28-day cycle

Remember: you don't ovulate when you are on the pill or using other hormonal birth control, so you won't be able to harness the benefits of cycle-syncing.

1

Feeling: tender, slow, reclusive, quiet, tired.

Time to: rest, retreat, go inwards, delegate your to-do list, eat nourishing pre-cooked meals, drink warming teas.

Exercise: gentle activities such as walking, stretching, yin yoga, plus meditation and breathwork.

2

Feeling: energetic, ego-driven, achievement-oriented.

Time to: start new projects, tackle your to-do list, read and learn, plan meetings, focus more on work and less on socialising; be mindful of your people skills as you can be more aggressive during this yang/masculine phase.

Exercise: strength and stamina exercises such as HIIT, power yoga, weights, resistance and jogging.

3

Feeling: energised, expressive, confident, fertile and horny; desire to hold and be held; nurturing, mother energy.

Time to: reconnect, socialise with your community, connect to your femininity by practising self-care including body or breast massage, go on dates with your partner or friends.

Exercise: continue with higher intensity exercise much like the follicular phase, but mix things up such as swapping running for cycling and weights for boxing.

4

Feeling: reflective, intuitive and creative, increased sensitivity of emotions and body.

Time to: declutter, finish projects, take time for self, such as soaking in a magnesium bath to replenish stores before period, reading, walking in nature, watching uplifting TV shows.

Exercise: incorporate a combination of high intensity and gentle exercise to reflect your changing mood.

Recommended apps: Menstrual tracking apps help you record your cyclical symptoms every month and also help you to track where in your cycle you will be at any given point in time. We love MyFLO, Moody, Clue and Flo.

While apps are wonderful for tracking your cycle and planning your weeks, they should not be treated as gospel, especially regarding ovulation. When tracking your fertility, we highly recommend checking your basal body temperature and cervical mucus throughout your cycle.

Recommended reading: *Blood Rites* by Jane Hardwicke Collings; *Period Power* by Maisie Hill; *In the Flo* by Alisa Vitti; *The Fifth Vital Sign* by Lisa Hendrickson-Jack.

SLEEP, OR LACK THEREOF

On average, new mothers lose 700 hours of sleep in the first year of their baby's life. In a society that measures success on how well your baby sleeps through the night, it can be hard not to feel like you are failing when your baby wants to be attached to your boob (or simply gazing at you as they babble away), all night, every night.

Parents have been known to do clumsy and unsafe things due to sleep deprivation. Leaving the keys in the front door is a popular one, as is almost falling asleep at the wheel or forgetting to turn off the stove. Something less openly discussed is that sleep deprivation can cause resentment, irritability, anger and rage, which can come as a shock to those of us who never experienced those feelings before.

While we can't help with baby's frequent waking (which, by the way, is biologically normal and developmentally important), we do have some tips on how to manage parental sleep deprivation.

Restorative Rest

Sleepless nights and long days with your baby can take their toll on your body and brain, and longstanding sleep deprivation puts parents at risk of both physical and mental health issues. When possible (and we know it's not always going to be), try to nap when your baby naps. This may only be for 15 minutes, once or twice per week, but every small amount of rest for your brain provides a multitude of benefits for your overall health.

If you are unable to sleep while your baby sleeps, resting while your baby sleeps is the next best thing. Lowering the lights and laying on the bed or couch near your baby, or on the floor with your legs up the wall can be incredibly therapeutic and restful if you allow yourself the time and space to do so. Stanford neuroscientist and researcher Dr Andrew Huberman recommends practising restorative rest, such as doing guided meditation, breathwork or yoga nidra, which helps us to focus less on our busy mind, and more on our body. These practices activate the parasympathetic nervous system and reduce stress hormones, including adrenaline and cortisol.

Tag Team

Whether it's sleeping in after tending to your baby all night, or taking the night in shifts, come up with a way that your partner can support you that works for your unique family constellation. Some partners get up early after the baby's morning feed, allowing mum to sleep until they have to go to work, or until the baby's next feed. (Brownie points if you return the baby with breakfast and tea/coffee for mama.)

Other families have an agreement where one parent handles bedtime until 2 am and the other handles 2 am until morning, or they alternate night on/night off. Some parents do the night shifts together, with one feeding and the other burping/changing and settling.

Of course this will be different again if you have multiple children who are waking through the night, and you may find yourself sleeping in one room with your baby, while your partner sleeps in another room with your other kiddos. Know that this is normal and families all around the world are doing the same thing. Whatever you can do to maximise sleep, do it!

Alternatively, Take a Reverse Sleep-In

Popularised by our friend Naomi Chrisoulakis, a reverse sleep-in is another way of saying early night. It involves going to bed very early to catch up on the hours of sleep you miss during the night. Naomi swears by doing this at least two nights a week, and has started a small revolution with other mothers in our community who now rely on this simple but genius idea to stay on top of sleep debt.

Let the Sunshine In

Modern humans spend an absurd amount of time indoors. While inside light provides few more benefits than improved eyesight, the natural beauty of the sun activates a number of hormones and health benefits in your body by triggering certain areas in your retina.

Exposure to natural sunlight on your face, especially first thing in the morning, kickstarts the body's innate body clock and circadian rhythm which allows us to create therapeutic amounts of waking, sleeping and mood regulating hormones (cortisol, melatonin and serotonin). Providing our body with the benefits of sunlight every morning allows it to create a healthy pattern of energy production, sleep encouragement and overall mood enhancement.

Avoid Blue Light During Night-time Feeds

It's all good and well for us to say 'don't look at your phone while you're feeding your baby', but we know this isn't a reality for most people. Many parents need stimulation during night feeds to either stay awake or relieve the boredom and/or loneliness that can come from feeding for hours on end. Blue light from our phones and laptops is beneficial during the daytime as it boosts attention, however it also suppresses melatonin production, which is our natural 'sleep' hormone, meaning time spent on your phone while feeding can make it more difficult to fall back asleep with ease, even when you are tired. If you are able to relax with a podcast or audiobook in your ears, great. If you need something more stimulating to stop you nodding off and find yourself scrolling on your phone or tablet, you can download blue light blocking filters on your device and also buy blue light blocking glasses.

Practise Good Sleep Habits

Being aware of sleep hygiene will ensure that when sleep is available it is good quality and restorative. Here are some strategies to support better sleep patterns:

- Swap scrolling on your phone for reading a book or listening to a guided meditation to reduce hyper-stimulation and allow your body to wind down.
- For dinner, eat a quality meal containing protein, healthy fats and complex carbohydrates to regulate blood sugar throughout the night.
- Avoid drinks such as caffeinated tea, coffee and soft drinks after 2 pm and opt for a chamomile, lemon balm or sleepy tea in the evening.
- A magnesium supplement (glycinate is best) can support your body to create and regulate 'GABA' – a neurotransmitter that supports the reduction of anxiety and sleep disturbances. It also supports the relaxation of muscles to reduce physical feelings of tension and restless legs, helping you drift off more easily.

Hot Tip for Tough Moments:

Have an agreement that nothing that gets said between you and your partner in the middle of the night counts. You are likely to call them a f*cking c*nt on more than one occasion, either because nothing they are trying to do is helping, or because they are snoring in ignorant bliss while you nurse your baby for hours on end. In some homes, this may even (need to) extend to 'nothing that gets said before my morning coffee counts'.

Remember, it's a Season

It can be hard not to get carried away with the intensity of sleep deprivation, especially when you've got half of society asking if your baby is sleeping through the night yet and the other reminding you that it's normal and you can expect to be tired for the next few years of their life. Argghhh!

In these moments, remember, everything is a season. Every season has beautiful parts and difficult parts. It can be tricky to not get caught up in the relentlessness of it all, whether it's sleeplessness, clinginess, or eating the dog biscuits. When you're in the thick of it, remind yourself that 'this too shall pass' and if you can, look at the situation from your child's point of view. Reframing the situation will prevent you from taking the behaviours of your child so personally, and arm you with the tools to help them. Perspective is EVERYTHING.

Meaningless Lists for Racing Minds:

When you want to sleep but are being kept awake by racing thoughts, there are a number of techniques you can use to create calm and quiet in your mind. One of our favourites is the use of meaningless lists.

Start with a theme – it may be an everyday theme, such as baby names, produce or animals, or it may be something more specific to your field of interest, such as films, books, plants, artists or athletes.

Go through the alphabet, thinking of two or three things for each letter – for example, Apple, Apricot, Avocado, Banana, Broccoli, Beans, Carrot, Cabbage, Capsicum and so on. If you get stuck on a letter, simply skip it and carry on.

You might get interrupted by a baby or a thought prompted by one of the words on your list that causes another stream of racing thoughts. When you notice this has happened, simply pick another letter and start again.

A Note on Sleep Training

Of all the topics in parenthood, sleep training might just be the most contentious. We live in a world where normal infant sleep has been pathologised, and from the moment they are born, we are asked how our babies are sleeping. While it is normal for babies and children to wake multiple times through the night until they are three to four years old, there are very few support systems for those who tend to these tiny, wakeful humans. As such, infant sleep is a multibillion-dollar industry with books, consultants, courses and gadgets dedicated to achieving the holy grail of parenting – a baby who sleeps through the night.

We understand the need for sleep, especially when you must return to work or when your mental health is waning due to sleep deprivation. If your family is struggling with sleep deprivation and you wish to seek out the assistance of a sleep consultant, we encourage the guidance of a qualified holistic sleep coach or specialist, who will take into account the developmental stage of your baby and your family dynamic. They will also assess the sleeping arrangements, psychological and emotional needs of everyone in the family and come up with an individualised plan that you can take at your own pace, honouring you as the true expert of your own baby. They will teach you about things such as sleep associations and how to see your child's cries as a means of communication, not manipulation. There is no one-size-fits-all solution, therefore the right holistic guide will support you through the many shades of grey until you find an approach that fits your family.

P.S. Don't worry, most people we know can't put their babies down 'drowsy but awake' either.

P.P.S. None of what we share here is meant to shame or judge, but rather provide you with all the info so you can make an informed decision about how to tackle your child's sleep.

'The "cry it out" approach seems to have arisen as a solution to the dissolution of extended family life in the 20th century. The vast knowledge of (now great, great) grandmothers was lost in the distance between households with children and those with the experience and expertise about how to raise them well. The wisdom of keeping babies happy was lost between generations.'

DARCIA NARVAEZ, PHD

MOOD SHIFTERS

We've already discussed the importance of exercise, but we wanted to take a moment to mention all the other ways you can shift your mood when you're exhausted or in a funk.

MOVEMENT

This can be a few light stretches, a walk around the block or a boogie to your favourite song. Whatever you choose, movement gets you out of your head and into your body. It releases stagnant energy and encourages the production of endorphins – chemical messengers that promote feelings of wellbeing and pleasure, while reducing feelings of pain and discomfort.

MUSIC

The benefits of musical therapy have been witnessed in various cultures for eons. Music has the ability to reduce anxiety and depression and increase wellbeing. For you, this might involve playing an instrument or listening to your favourite artist or playlist. Be selective of the volume and pace and turn it up or down depending on whether you need grounding or a boost.

NATURE AND FRESH AIR

For both mothers and their children, stepping outside for some space and fresh air can do serious wonders for the nervous system. Studies have shown that when people spend time outdoors, especially in nature and green spaces, it improves memory and attention span, while decreasing mental distress. 'Biophilia' is the innate drive to connect with nature and other living beings. This is backed up by stress reduction and attention restoration theories, which indicate that time spent outdoors lowers stress and restores concentration.

WATER

Both cold and warm water immersion has noted benefits for supporting the nervous system and reducing stress, due to its ability to reduce stress hormones, including cortisol and adrenaline, while relaxing muscles and reducing pain.

RITUAL

Whether you know it or not, you probably have lots of rituals you observe throughout your day. From preparing your first cup of tea in the silence of the morning to layering on your favourite skincare before hopping into bed at night, rituals can make you feel calm and grounded in a time when the rest of your world feels out of control. They don't need to be 'woo-woo', they simply (but oh-so-powerfully) bring meaning and purpose when life feels otherwise mundane. Some other examples include journalling, lighting a candle, diffusing essential oils, soaking in a warm bath, pulling tarot cards, or listening to a guided meditation.

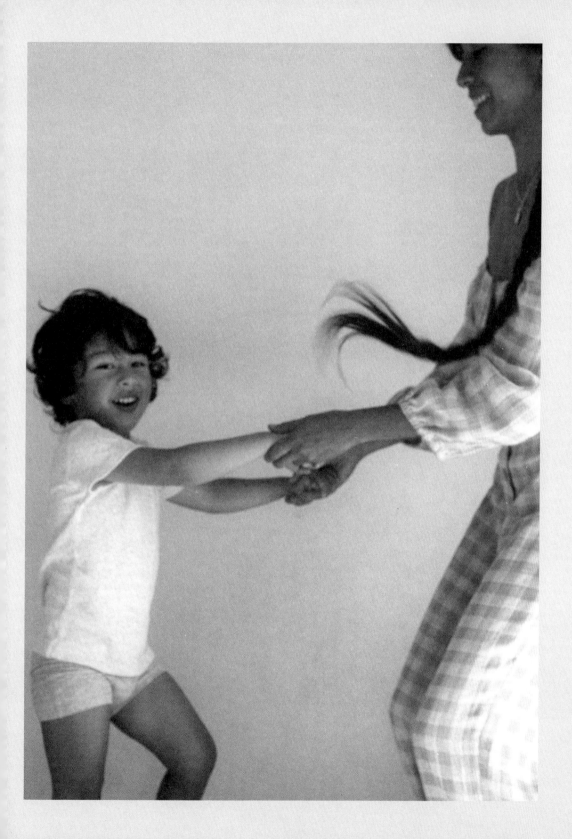

A Note on the Vagus Nerve

The vagus nerve is a long, wandering nerve pathway that originates at the medulla oblongata portion of the brain stem and branches through tissues and organs found in the face, neck, chest and abdomen – including the vocal cords, digestive tract, heart and lungs, liver, spleen and kidneys, amongst others.

This network of sensory and motor fibres creates communication between the brain, the nervous system and the gut – carrying important information back to the brain about what is going on in the body, while regulating subconscious bodily functions such as swallowing, breathing, heart rate, alertness, arousal, immune function and digestion. Most importantly, the vagus nerve is involved in the regulation of the parasympathetic nervous system – or 'rest and digest' function of the body, which helps to calm us down and counterpoint the sympathetic nervous system during times of stress and 'fight or flight' response.

'Vagal tone' is a biological process that is determined by the activity of the vagus nerve, with strong vagal tone being the result of a positive feedback loop between good physical health and emotional state, and activation of the parasympathetic nervous system which promotes adaptation and relaxation after a state of stress. Weak vagal tone is associated with poor physical and emotional health, and often occurs as a result of long term, chronic stress. Studies have shown that it is linked to a number of health concerns including anxiety, mood disorders, insomnia, chronic pain, digestive issues and cardiovascular disease, amongst others.

Research has also shown that vagal tone can be passed from mother to infant, with mothers who are anxious, depressed or angry having weaker vagal tone than those without mood concerns, and following birth, their newborns also having reduced vagal activity and lower levels of serotonin and dopamine.

The good news is that the vagus nerve can be toned and strengthened through a number of practices, which can be easily incorporated into your daily life to improve overall physical and mental health. Science continues to better understand and promote activities that encourage a strong vagal tone, which include spending time in nature, breathwork, cold showers, mindfulness and meditation, laughter, gargling and singing/humming, nostril breathing and supporting optimal digestive health with specific wholefoods and supplements.

There is a growing number of evidence-based information available on supporting the health of your vagus nerve, which we highly encourage you to investigate to support your own wellbeing on the parenthood journey.

Vagus Nerve Tip:

If you are experiencing feelings of overwhelm or rage while holding your baby (and you feel in a good enough headspace to keep holding them), try humming out loud to soothe your nervous system. The vagus nerve travels through the vocal cords, which studies have shown both humming and singing to activate and tone. Not only can this practice support your own vagal health, but also your baby's nervous system by regulating their levels of stress hormones that are so sensitive and in tune with your own.

Nervous System Support Tools

What can you do for yourself when you aren't feeling your best? It is important to identify exactly what you are feeling in order to know which steps to take to improve your mental state. The thought of physically doing something may feel overwhelming, but it's important to understand you are bigger than your emotions, and the ability to change them lies within taking simple but potent action.

IF YOU ARE FEELING WIRED, ANXIOUS, WORKED UP OR ON EDGE, CHOOSE AN ACTIVITY THAT IS SOOTHING.

- Calming music
- Warm bath
- Aromatherapy: lavender, sweet orange, chamomile
- Foot soak
- Face mask
- Journalling
- Drawing or painting
- Meditation
- Breathwork
- Lighting a candle
- Oil massage
- Walking near the ocean or a river

IF YOU ARE FEELING FLAT, FATIGUED, DISCONNECTED, SAD OR UNMOTIVATED, START WITH GENTLE ACTIVITIES THAT ARE ACTIVATING.

- Cooking
- Gardening
- Energising music
- Having a boogie
- Calling a friend
- Cold shower
- Going out for coffee or lunch
- Walking or jogging
- Cleaning
- Breathwork

NAVIGATING FAMILY LIFE

As we discussed in chapter one, your relationship with your partner has undoubtedly changed.

Some couples find themselves in a love bubble, utterly smitten with this miracle they have created. Others find themselves overwhelmed with resentment and rage because their life has changed so inexplicably while their partner's life remains seemingly unchanged. Almost every couple we know has been at both ends of the spectrum, and we want you to know it is completely normal to find yourself fantasising about leaving your partner (and for this to be the only fantasy you have about them for the first few weeks or months of your baby's life).

The latter is usually a response to an extreme amount of stress and severe lack of sleep, validation and support. Exhaustion and stress are the undoing of even the most solid foundations and it is often in those early and sleepless days of parenthood that even the most compatible people realise how incompatible their stress responses are.

It is common for the birthing person to be so focused on the survival of her baby for the first two years of its life that she is emotionally and energetically unable to provide for the needs of her partner. If you are feeling adrift from your partner, it may be worth revisiting the relationships section in chapter one (starting on page 27), tuning into each other's Love Languages™, and utilising the 'the story in my head is' tool to communicate your feelings in a neutral way.

Here are some tips for dividing the physical and mental load of raising a family:

- Work with your strengths. One of you may be good at paying bills, doing laundry and cleaning whereas the other may be good at cooking, managing appointments and tidying.
- Communicate! There is so much that goes into raising happy and healthy little humans, and the mental load can be crippling at times. If you feel like you are taking on more than your partner, a discussion about all the things you have to think about in a day might be in order. While we want our partners to be mind-readers, they aren't.
- View it as 'the load' rather than 'mine vs. yours'. It's easy to be so consumed by your own load that you forget how hard the other person is working. This is where resentment kicks in. By viewing it as 'the load' rather than 'mine vs. yours', you are more likely to act as a team.
- Relax your standards a little. Things aren't going to be like this forever. Of course, if having a tidy home is important for your sanity, then having a tidy home should be prioritised. Figure out what your priorities are and what you feel is okay to let slide.
- Have a list. When you both have a clear view of all that needs to be achieved in a day, week or month, it can make the division seem easier.
- Remember, being home with a newborn is a FULL-TIME JOB. Feeding alone takes up more than thirty hours a week. Just because you are home all day does not mean you should be the only one taking care of all of the household chores. One partner goes to work, the other stays home with a baby. Everything else in the household should be split.

IN CASE YOU NEED A LITTLE HELP COMMUNICATING WE ASKED SOME MOTHERS IN OUR COMMUNITY WHAT MAKES UP THEIR MENTAL LOAD. HERE'S WHAT THEY CAME BACK WITH:

'In no particular order ... Admin related to all enrolments, due dates, vaccinations, payments for any lessons e.g. music, swimming etc.; upcoming friends' birthdays and presents; cleaning out and recycling outgrown clothes, shoes and toys; researching ideas for play that isn't TV; researching (and shopping for) meals that hide vegetables; researching and learning about strategies for facilitating upcoming socially expected milestones e.g. sleep, toilet training, starting school etc. Worrying about how to respond to challenging behaviour e.g. hitting, not listening etc.; researching and listening to experts on these topics ... Um probably forgetting a billion other things due to the mental load itself frying me out.' – Emily Hehir

'Food. So much food. Preparing and making. Planning. Buying. Cleaning. Cooking. Serving. Drink bottles ... cleaning them, filling them. Reminding them to drink water. Snacks (making and offering). Vitamins. Naps. Timing outings for naps (toddler) and watching for tired signs (baby). Nail cutting. Hair cutting. Clothes – buying and organising plus rearranging every time they grow (regularly). Thinking and buying ahead. Spending hours finding the clothes that aren't contributing to landfill, aren't awful but are affordable. Sunscreen and sun protection. Etc. etc. etc.' – Amy Pearson

'ALL of the above, plus: Have I read them enough books, done enough stimulating play, given them enough "free play" to develop their own imagination and creative play? Do they sleep enough? Snore too much? Fit in with their friends? Assert themselves enough or are they too bossy? Do we send them to kinder or hold them back? Have I spoken to them enough about social injustices or have I spoiled their innocence too early? Are their favourite clothes washed and dry for day care or is this going to lead to mega meltdowns tomorrow morning? Are the clothes they wear 'gender neutral' enough? Or am I going to be judged for dressing them in frills that they were gifted? Did I put on sunscreen and an extra layer of zinc for the beach? Is the sunscreen all natural? Which sleeping bag do I pack to make sure they are not too hot or too cold while on holidays? Should I post this pic on social media or am I ruining their privacy? How long are we going to be out for, how many snacks and drinks do I need? Are they healthy enough? What weird insecurities and idiosyncrasies am I unknowingly passing onto them? Do we spend enough time in nature? Are we up to date with immunisations and invoices?' – Rowie Cooke

LET'S TALK ABOUT SEX AFTER BABY

This is a biggie.

The recommended wait time from health professionals between giving birth and intercourse is four to six weeks to allow vaginal or vulvar injuries to heal, lochia discharge to ease and to minimise risk of infection. But when we asked the mothers in our community about their sex life after birth, the results were incredibly varied. While there was a large cluster who waited between four to six months before having sex for the first time, there were others who waited much longer than this (and some who could barely wait at all). Many admitted to feelings of shame about how long it took them to have sex and about how much their sex life had changed now they are parents.

Dr Martien Snellen says in his book *Rekindling*, 'The postpartum period is generally a time of transition, and it isn't unusual for this to affect the nature and frequency of a couple's sex life, if pregnancy hasn't already altered it irrevocably. It's a complicated business involving social and cultural influences, physical changes, an altered emotional state, contextual factors, breastfeeding, relational changes, loss of autonomy, changes in body- and self-image and the process of psychologically adjusting to parenthood – not to mention good old-fashioned exhaustion.'

Regardless of how long we wait before resuming intercourse, our sex life changes drastically for most of us after we have kids, and it can take months (and even years) for your sex drive and emotional state to feel truly ready. Following birth, your hormones are focused on breastfeeding and recovery, rather than libido, with the lactation hormone prolactin counteracting arousal and low levels of oestrogen often causing vaginal dryness. The style of sex you enjoyed before giving birth might not feel good anymore or may even feel painful. For many who have been conditioned to believe sex is an act of giving and partner pleasing, the thought of offering your body and energy on top of all you give as a new mother can feel suffocating.

Hormones, physical trauma or injury from birth, exhaustion, being touched out, feeling like our body now belongs to our baby, resentment (whether conscious or subconscious) towards our partner for seemingly how little their life has changed, all come into play here. In addition, many of us don't realise until we fall pregnant that sex often took place after a wine or three, and we feel embarrassed talking about our needs without the disinhibition of alcohol and other substances. Many close confidantes have said they feel more comfortable telling a one night stand what they want in bed than their partner of ten years.

We live in a world where a healthy sex life is seen as the holy grail in a relationship, but what about security, contentment, shared goals and making each other laugh until you cry? Does physical repulsion at the thought of having sex matter if your relationship is perfect in every other way? Ultimately, that depends on you and your partner; when there is a disparity in the sexual needs of each person in a relationship, it's important to work on staying connected so you can ensure both of your needs are being met.

'Today we turn to one person to provide what an entire village once did: a sense of grounding, meaning and continuity. At the same time, we expect our committed relationships to be romantic as well as emotionally and sexually fulfilling. Is it any wonder that so many relationships crumble under the weight of it all? It's hard to generate excitement, anticipation and lust with the same person you look to for comfort and stability, but it's not impossible. For some of us, love and desire are inseparable. But for many others, emotional intimacy inhibits erotic expression.'

ESTHER PEREL, *MATING IN CAPTIVITY*

Staying Connected

Every interaction with your partner is an opportunity for connection. How do you react when they speak to or share something with you? Do you put your phone down, look up from your baby, pay attention to what they are saying and respond, or do you continue what you are doing and dismiss them?

Dr John Gottman refers to these moments as 'bids' and our reactions to them as either 'turning towards' or 'turning away'. In his research he found that couples whose marriages lasted turned towards each other 86 per cent of the time and couples who ended up divorced or separated turned towards each other only 33 per cent of the time.

It is important to carve out uninterrupted connection time with your partner. We know, we know, you hear this everywhere, but date nights are a great place to begin, even if they happen in the comfort of your own home. It is more than understandable that the idea of leaving your child/ren with someone else may induce anxiety or be logistically difficult, but if and when possible, it can be beneficial for you as a couple to get out of the house together and shift away from the monotony of parenthood. If a date night is out of the question, try having lunch in the park or even a takeaway coffee and a walk around the block.

Planned Intimacy

Euphemia Russell, full spectrum pleasure coach and bestselling author of *Slow Pleasure* says, 'As a culture, we're obsessed with thinking that authentic intimacy needs to be spontaneous. Yet, with anything that is important to you in your life you plan it so you can prioritise it, and carve out space for deep attention and presence.

I suggest to literally everyone in relationships that you plan pleasure time. That doesn't mean sexual pleasure and scheduling sex, but rather body-focused pleasure together like massages, baths, holding hands and going for a walk to look at details, making out, taking sexy photos of each other, whatever feels enlivening for both/all of you.

See it as an opportunity to mutually soften, open, and deepen with each other amongst the chaos of life with children.

It's also important that if you're sexually intimate that there isn't pressure to always escalate the intensity of that dynamic. So if you are making out, release expectation that it will escalate to a particular type of sexual pleasure. Practise seeing pleasure as meandering, non-goal oriented, and non-hierarchical.'

Tips for Partners:

It may take a long time before your partner has any semblance of a libido after giving birth. Be patient, and when they are ready take it slow and gentle. Even if your partner has been given the thumbs up by their GP, they may not feel physically or emotionally ready. Let them take the lead and read their facial cues to see if they are enjoying it or not. Use lots of lube, take lots of breaks, and don't be alarmed if they spray breastmilk on you – this can happen during an orgasm.

Lube It Up!

When you are ready for your sex life to resume, start slow and remember, lube is your friend. Not all lubricants are created equal and many over the counter or supermarket brands can contain parabens and other nasty ingredients that may disrupt your vaginal microbiome and increase risk of infections. It's smart to stay away from flavoured lubes as these contain sugars which may throw your vaginal pH out of balance, and avoid any containing glycerin, which despite its short term benefits, can actually pull moisture out of your vaginal tissue. A good rule of thumb is to choose a natural, water-based lubricant or play around with organic, unrefined plant oils such as coconut or jojoba oil. If using a condom it's important to note that oils can break down natural latex, causing condoms to tear. If you do experience any discomfort while using these, keep playing around until you find something that works.

A Word About Porn

We are living in a time where all and any type of porn is available at the click of a button, and for that reason it's important we are informed and are able to have non-judgemental, shame-free conversations about it. If your partner is viewing porn as an outlet for their unmet sexual needs, you may be deeply disturbed (if you see it as a type of infidelity), or you may see it as a relief (as your partner jacking off to porn frees you from sexual 'obligations'). Regardless of where you sit with it, frequent porn consumption is dangerous because it can literally rewire the brain.

The visually stimulating properties of porn make it a powerful trigger for the brain. A common comparison by scientists is that of porn consumption and substance abuse, due to them both creating surges in dopamine – the feel-good and reward neurotransmitter. This neurotransmitter plays an important role in programming memories and information. Therefore, when the body is seeking something like sexual pleasure, it remembers where to go to experience those same feelings and rewards.

The intensity of porn, much like that of highly addictive substances, causes an unnaturally high level of dopamine secretion. When watched often and repeatedly, porn can damage the dopamine reward system and cause it to be unresponsive or apathetic to more natural sources of pleasure which, over time, may lead to difficulty in becoming aroused with your partner. This is where porn can take the place of turning to a romantic partner to fulfil sexual desires and pleasures. Simply turning on a phone or laptop can become more accessible and instantly gratifying than taking the time and effort to turn on a partner.

That being said, if watching porn together is a way for you and your partner to get in the mood – great! We respect and encourage all types of sexual exploration, provided all involved parties feel respected and comfortable.

Make the Most of Daytime Sex:

If you are too exhausted for sex by the time your children are finally asleep at night, try getting jiggy with it during nap time instead. Many of the mothers in our community swear by this for keeping their connection alive.

FINDING YOUR VILLAGE

We hear 'it takes a village to raise a child' but rarely are we told how that village is built, where to find it, or what it looks like. So by now, you may be wondering where the f*ck that ever-elusive village is. When we become parents, we realise that the friends and family we thought were our village are busy people with busy lives, and just because our world has changed doesn't mean theirs can too.

If you were part of a tight friendship circle and are the first to have a baby, the experience can be alienating. In times of loneliness, remember, there are over 300,000 babies born every day worldwide. Somewhere, out there, there are people just like you; you just have to find them.

You may be surprised at the new friendships that blossom and old friendships that rekindle when you have a baby. Building a village with intention takes work and requires vulnerability. It requires you to reach out to strangers, acquaintances, and friends of friends. It can be scary, awkward and clumsy. Sometimes you won't vibe with a person as well as you thought you would, and other times you might really like each other but your kids hate each other.

Our advice is to keep searching. Trust that you will find a person who makes you feel at ease when you are together. Someone you can invite over when your house is at its messiest, and when you're an un-showered, milk-stained mess. There will be a person you can drink endless cups of tea with while you fold laundry, and who can hold your baby while you cook, and someone whose kids can play with yours while you clean your kitchen. A friend whose mere presence makes the load of parenthood and domesticity lighter. These friendships may see you through a lifetime or a season. What's important is that you feel held, seen and supported through one of the most beautiful, intense and brutal times of your life.

There is also something to be said about the global community. While the village may be all but lost (for now), we are lucky to live in an age where technology connects us to friends, lactation consultants, psychologists, doulas and sleep experts all over the world. While online exchanges don't compare to real-life ones, they provide connection in what can be a very lonely time.

Outgrowing Friendships

Your postpartum is a good time to shed friendships that you have outgrown or that are no longer serving you. This can be hard, but the relief is worth it. It's incredible to look back on how much you used to tolerate, when your heart wasn't so tender and when you could carry the burden of obligation because your energy wasn't so precious. By making peace with relationships that no longer serve us, we create more space and time for positivity and growth.

Friendship breakups need not be dramatic. They can happen gently and honestly, probably with tears but hopefully with a lot of deep breaths and relief, and not too much drama. In saying that, hurt or drama can force us to evaluate the integrity of a relationship, or give us the courage to end one. When working through resentments, it's important to keep in mind that forgiveness does not require reconnection, and you can forgive without reconciliation.

About those resentments and grudges, we love the Buddhist thinking that says 'Holding onto anger is like drinking poison and expecting the other person to die'. When you are a mother, it is even more pertinent. Our children's nervous systems are so deeply attuned to ours that when we hold onto negativity it affects them too.

With everything we have to deal with, we deserve friendships where we are celebrated. Friends who feel like rest. Friends who build us up, speak highly of us, support us without judgement, remain curious when we hold an opposing opinion on something, and most of all, who we can be our authentic selves with. Life, and especially life once you become a parent, can be really, really hard. Friendships shouldn't be.

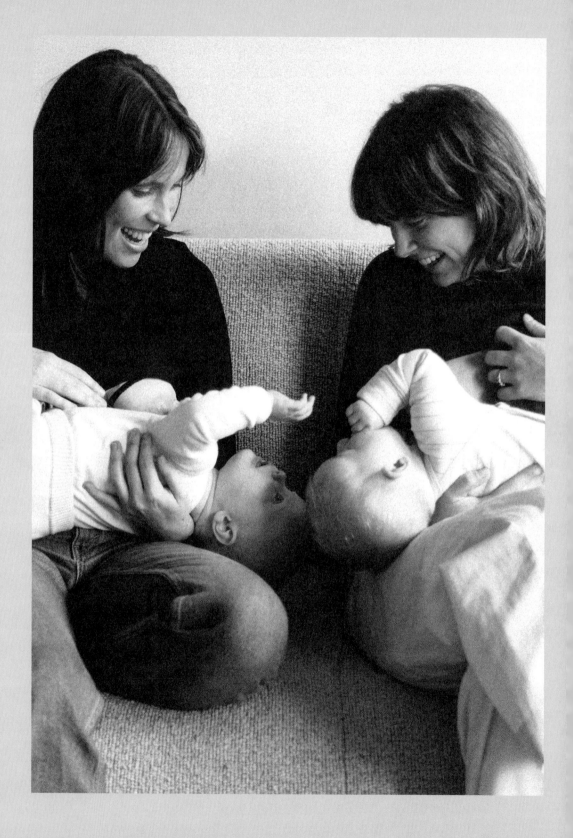

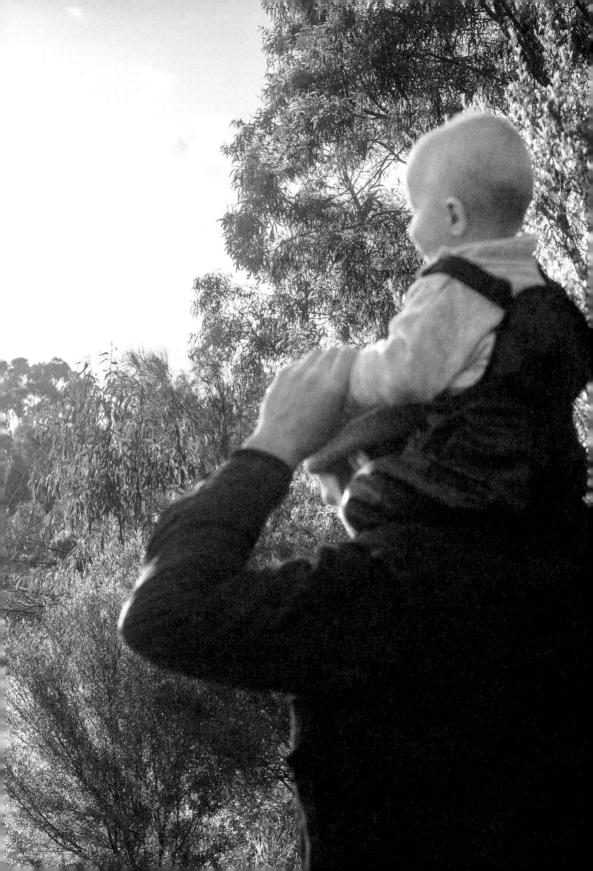

BIG LITTLE EMOTIONS

Parenting. It's Intense, Huh!

For a start, it's relentless. The emotions are HUGE, and no matter how much of yourself you give, it never seems to be enough. Perhaps one of the most shocking things about parenthood is the difference between expectations and reality. It's rare that parenthood looks, feels or rewards in the way we imagined, and it's even rarer that our children are who we thought they would be. Not only that, but no two children are ever the same, which can be a shock when we think we've got things all figured out and then a new one comes along and throws a spanner in the works.

This can be difficult to appreciate when you're in the trenches of a sleep regression or weighed down by the mind-numbing monotony of parenthood, but children really are our greatest teachers. Every one of them is a tiny mirror, reflecting our most wonderful qualities and worst habits. They also highlight the areas where your own inner child has an unhealed need for love and attention.

You Are Their Safe Place

When you're in the thick of it, it can help to remember that you are your child's safe place. Children hold everything inside until they feel safe to let it out with the person they feel most comfortable with, and that's you! You are the person who has been responsible for regulating their nervous system since the day they arrived on this planet and it can help to remember that when they are reacting to the wrong coloured fork or their toast being cut into little triangles instead of big triangles. Their reaction usually has nothing to do with the fork or the toast, but rather it is related to their need to recalibrate after the inevitable overstimulation that comes from being a curious little human who is absorbing absolutely everything around them. In fact, they may even ask for something they know you are going to say no to, because they are seeking an emotional release in order to feel regulated again.

If big emotions were not tolerated in your home growing up, it may be difficult for you to remain calm when your child experiences them. When they are having a release, what is most beneficial for them is for you to demonstrate the emotional regulation tools we discussed back in chapter one (page 23). Your child needs you to hold them with compassion and validate their (very real to them) problem. Diminishing or invalidating their experience, or punishing them for their behaviour (which they have no control over, by the way) only makes them feel unseen, unheard and inhibits their ability to learn how to regulate their emotions.

> **Kids Crave Consistency:**
>
> At times when things are outside their usual rhythm such as Christmas, school holidays or trips away, children can experience big emotions because they struggle to cope with the unpredictability. Consider that your toddler isn't being difficult, but rather they are having a difficult time.

Coping with Mess

The same goes for mess. People who grew up in homes where mess was not tolerated may often have trouble remaining calm as their toddlers tear through the home like a hurricane, leaving a trail of mass destruction in their wake. If this is you, then whenever you find yourself getting overwhelmed by the chaos, stop and take a breath. Your worth is not linked to the tidiness of your home. Cleaning up after one activity before starting the next is a great habit to cultivate, but children are still going to trash the place at times. If you can, make cleaning up a fun game and it will soon turn into an activity your children love.

Reconnection and Repair

If taking responsibility and apologising wasn't modelled to you by your caregivers this could be another challenging area when you become a parent. It's okay if you don't get it right every time, no one does. We all mess up, often multiple times per day. The most important thing we can do after we lose our shit is attempt what we call the 'reconnection and repair' phase. By taking accountability for our mistakes we model to our children how to repair their own moments of dysregulation.

This is important not only when our children are walking, talking, tiny tornadoes, but when they are babies too. If you're not good at owning your mistakes and apologising in your adult relationships, babies and children are wonderful people to practise this on, because they will never judge or laugh at you; they will only respond with love.

Tips to Repair After Losing Your Sh!t:

Get on their level: Squat down, sit on the floor, or lay on their bed with them and position your body so you can make eye contact. Get close enough that you can pull them in for a cuddle if they are ready to do so.

Apologise: Learn to say, 'I'm sorry for upsetting you.'

Acknowledge what happened: From a place of sincerity, relay what happened to your child. It can be as simple as 'I got cross and I yelled.'

Remind them that you love them: 'I love you so much and I don't like making you sad.'

Tell them you will do better next time: 'I will try not to yell next time I have big feelings.'

Hug it out: But be mindful whether they are ready to do so.

Reflect: Think about what's going on for you that led to the outburst. What can you do in order to be able to regulate your emotions next time parenting gets too much? When we tend to our children from a resourced place we are showing them the best versions of ourselves.

Recommended resource: Big Little Feelings have an online course that we recommend for anyone who is lost or struggling with managing the big feelings of their little human.

CONNECTION THROUGH PLAY

Healthy connection with us is one of the key things our children crave. The way we connect with them during the first three years of their life sets the ground for our relationship with them, and their relationship with the world, for the rest of their life. Connection also releases hormones and chemicals that are important for brain development. The responsibility can seem crippling at times!

When our children are babies, we connect and form strong attachments by holding them, making lots of eye contact and tending to their needs. As they grow older their needs and demands change, and what they require from us will vary from day to day, and child to child. Play is one of the most important ways of connecting with your children, filling their cups, and making them feel like you are on their level.

Children don't have the ability to say 'I've had a hard day, can we talk?' Instead, they say 'Can you play with me?' Below are some ways to connect through play when your imagination is all dried up, you're exhausted, don't like playing, or you just have too much to do.

Get Outdoors

When you are having a hard day the thought of leaving the house can seem impossible, terrifying or both. Even on a good day, leaving the house with one or multiple children is a full-time job, but on days where one or all of you are in a funk, there is truly no better way to reset than getting outdoors.

This is especially true when you have an unfathomably long to-do list and your children just won't stop clinging to you or bickering. They sense our distraction which unsettles their nervous systems, causing them to seek out our attention through unwanted behaviour. It's an instinct! Getting outside and connecting them with nature is a powerful antidote to intensity. Remember how we spoke about the power of nature to reset our nervous systems? It's the same for our little ones. Even on a rainy day, putting on a jacket and gumboots and going for a walk around the block while you splash in puddles is a fun and hilarious activity that will fill their little cups. If you can make the time to do this, they will be happier to spend time by themselves when you get home, allowing you to tend to whatever pressing tasks await.

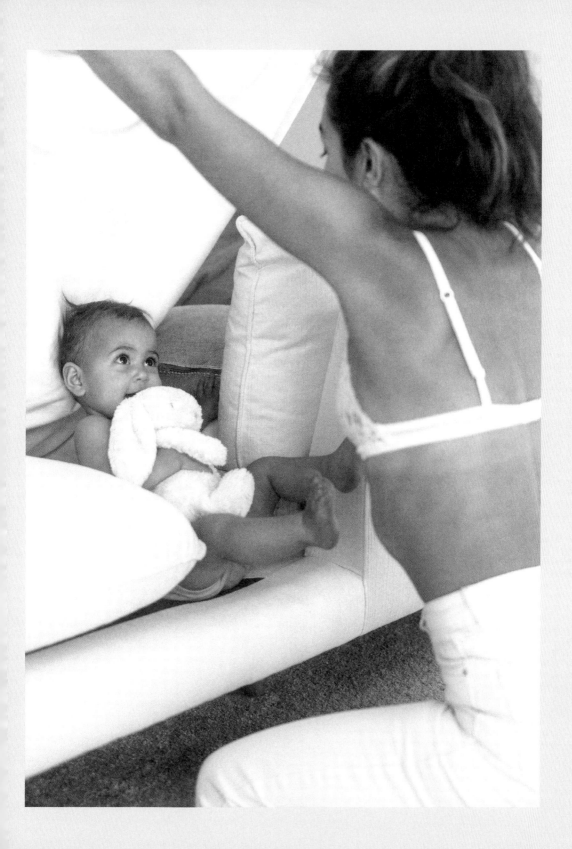

Sensory Play

While nature is an incredible source of sensory play, there are other options when you can't leave the house. Whether it be a vessel of water or a bowl of rice, sensory play is renowned for providing hours of fun and entertainment to our little ones. As well as building neural connections and helping them develop language and motor skills, it helps them regulate sensory stimuli, practise problem-solving, and be laser-focused on one task (which is the part that allows you to get sh*t done).

You can do this in the kitchen, keeping an eye on your child as you cook dinner, or set up a couple of different tubs that you can pull out when you need to tame a wildling while you tend to a younger child. Tubs can be filled with things like penne pasta and a ball of string, shells and gemstones hidden in kinetic sand, or hide a couple of diggers in a tub of rice – the options are limitless. Frequent op shops for things such as wooden bowls and scoopers and build a sensory play station over time.

Horizontal Play

When you are sick, exhausted, bleeding, or straight-up out of ideas, horizontal play is a lifesaver. Simply lay on the ground and let them lead, or suggest one of the following games if they need a little more stimulation:

What's on My Butt?? Is a game created by an anonymous mum and popularised by Hillary Frank. If you have small children, you can imagine their squeals of laughter as they place objects on your butt and you jiggle your butt-cheeks around while you try to guess what they are. This can also be played laying on your back or side. The aim of the game is to guess what object they have put on you. It's impossible to guess, which is wonderful for confidence building as children love when adults are wrong.

Ninjas involves setting up an obstacle course and then laying down with your eyes closed. The aim of the game is for your children to complete the course as quietly as possible. If you hear them you open your eyes and they have to go back to the start. Genius!

Other clever suggestions from our community are:

- Massage/Hair Salons/Doctors – you are always the client/patient, obviously.
- Draw Me Sleeping – the name says it all.
- Dead Fish/Sleeping Lions or any variation of, where the aim of the game is to stay still for the longest.
- Babies – you are the baby and the toddler is the parent.
- Blanketland/Pillowland – you lie down and get your kids to cover you in pillows or blankets.
- Lay on the grass and look at the cloud animals – a reminder that you can be outside and horizontal.
- Body Race Track – lay on the ground and let your child drive their cars all over you.

Let Them Be Bored

It's impossible to play with your children all day every day, so when they wander around the house saying they are bored, try not to feel guilty. Being bored is important for imagination because it allows time to rest and find an inward, quiet space which forces them to come up with creative ways to entertain themselves.

Just Add Water!

Ask any parent, and they will agree that water has the ability to magically transform a little human's mood. Not only is it soothing, but it entertains them for hours. Some ways to incorporate water when you need to calm your household a little:

- Fill your sink with soapy bubbles, pull up a learning tower, and give them some bowls and utensils to 'wash' – perfect for when you need to entertain little ones while you get started on dinner.
- Run a bath. If they don't want to get in, climb in yourself and they will probably want to join.
- Set up a towel on the floor and place a couple of bowls of water on it, along with some toy animals or jugs/spoons/scoops/funnels etc.
- Fill a spray bottle with water and get them to 'clean' the windows, floor, spray the side of the house, the fence, your outdoor plants etc.
- For outdoor water play, fill your paddling pool, turn on the sprinkler, or set up a water play table. Mud kitchens also provide endless hours of fun if you're game enough.
- If leaving the house is an option, trips to bodies of water such as lakes, rivers, the ocean and waterfalls. This also provides an opportunity to learn about our planet and all the beautiful creatures who inhabit it.

A reminder that babies and children should never be left alone with water. They can drown in as little as 5 cm (2 in), so while water play is often a relief on clingy, bossy or tantrumy days, it must always been done under supervision, and all water vessels should be emptied once water play has finished.

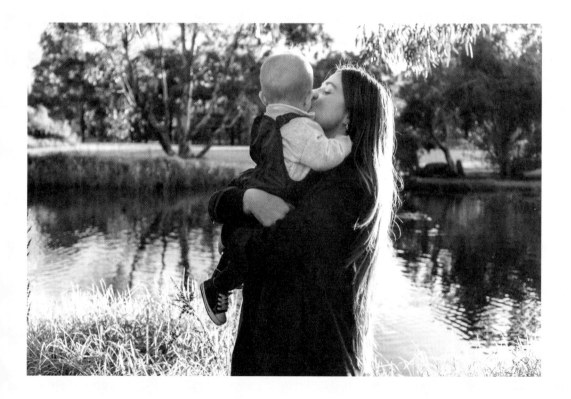

PRACTICAL TIPS FOR GETTING THROUGH THE DAY

How to Leave the House Like a Boss

No matter if you have one child or five, whether you're driving or walking, leaving the house can feel overwhelming and anxiety-inducing. Not only are there worries about how your baby will cope and what germs they will encounter, but there is also an unfathomable amount of organisation involved. Below are some tips (think of them as insurance policies) to help make trips out of the home a little bit easier.

BE ORGANISED

Gone are the days where you could simply grab your keys and go. Babies are notorious for sleeping or feeding for extra long periods of time when you have somewhere to be, or spewing (or pooing) all over themselves the moment you get in the car. Not to mention the toddlers who take fifteen hundred hours to put on their shoes ... The easiest way to avoid feeling rushed or stressed about getting out the door in time is to start the process a good 15–30 minutes before you plan to be reversing out your driveway. Shoes on, teeth brushed, nappy bag and everything else you're taking lined up at the door. Control the things you can, and expect the unexpected.

We recommend having a bag pre-packed with the following:

- Nappies and a change mat.
- Wipes (such a saviour for spills and sticky hands).
- Change of clothes.
- Hats and sunscreen.
- Toys. Pack a favourite plus one they haven't played with for a while for novelty factor. Sand toys if you're going to the beach or a playground and drawing materials if you're going to a cafe.
- Playmat or rug if going to a park or playground.
- Pram or carrier if you are going in the car but plan to get out and about.
- Lip balm and earplugs or whatever other creature comforts you need.
- A reusable coffee cup to enjoy a takeaway beverage.
- Snacks for you and the kids.
- Water bottle for you and the kids.

It can be helpful to have most of the bag packed and ready to go at all times, then just add water and snacks when you are ready to leave the house. Give it a once over in case something was removed and not put back in. There's nothing quite like dealing with a poo when you don't have any wipes.

> **Hot Tip:**
>
> Keep spare wipes, nappies and a beach towel in your car at all times; you never know when you will need it, but you will thank yourself when the time comes.

DRESS YOURSELF AT THE LAST POSSIBLE MINUTE

Whether this means knowing what you are going to wear and being in your undies until the moment you are about to walk out the door, or wearing a robe over your outfit until you've popped your kids in the stroller or car, this will prevent spew, poo and grubby hands forcing you into a last minute outfit change.

IF YOU CAN, FEED AND DO A NAPPY CHANGE BEFORE YOU LEAVE

A full baby with a dry bum is bound to be more content than a hungry and wet one.

AVOID PEAK HOUR OR CROWDED ANYTHING

Your first outing with a newborn will ideally be something short and close to home, such as a stroll around the block or a trip to visit a close friend in a neighbouring suburb. As your kids get older, consider if their little nervous systems can handle the outing. A trip to a park or grandparents' house – wonderful. A trip to the supermarket or shopping mall in peak hour traffic – recipe for disaster.

REMEMBER, IT'S OKAY IF YOUR BABY CRIES ...

... even if they don't usually cry at home. You don't need to feel shame, and you are not the world's worst parent. People generally expect babies to cry and anyone who is inconvenienced by this, well ... that's more about them than it is about you. Contrary to how you may feel, most people aren't looking on in horror while you fail to appease your small human, nor have they been crying for as long as you feel like they have.

On a positive note, we promise, leaving the house does get easier. At some point soon, you'll turn a corner and all of a sudden, they will be walking themselves to the car with a toy in one hand and no nappy in sight.

Deep Breaths

When your child is hurt or upset, help bring them back into their body by taking three deep breaths together. Teaching them to use their breath to regulate their nervous system is one of the greatest gifts you can give them. While they don't always understand or show interest in what you are teaching them, with time and repetition, your gentle guidance will eventually click. When it does, it becomes a grounding tool for them to draw on, even when you're not there to remind them. Taking deep breaths with your child can also help your own nervous system and reduce your own sense of overwhelm as you try to navigate their big little emotions.

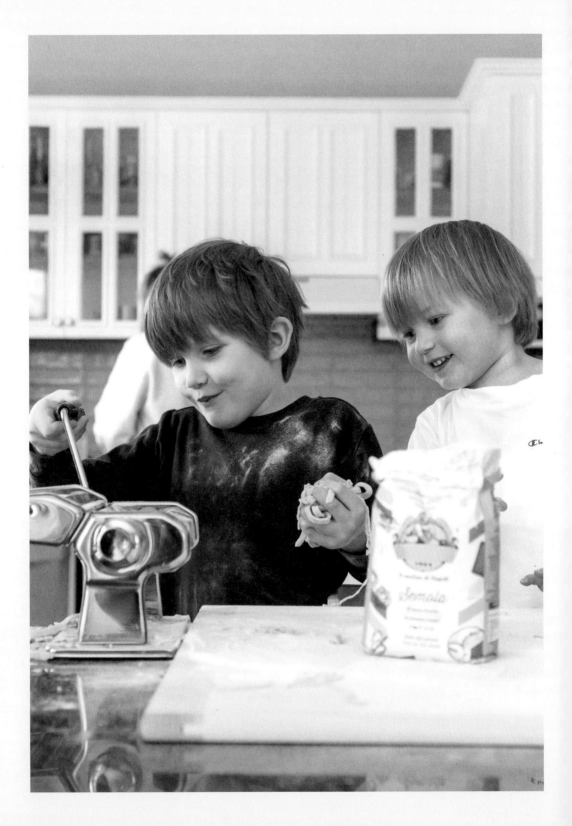

Managing Mealtimes

Food and mealtimes tend to be extremely stressful for parents. Making food takes time, makes mess, and then no one eats it anyway. Not only that, but nourishing yourself can be tricky on top of the demands of our little ones.

COOK MORE, LESS OFTEN

Meal planning and prepping doesn't work for everyone, and it can be difficult to pull off successfully when you have so much shit in your brain that you cannot possibly fit a list of groceries in there too. Having a few meals on rotation and making them every week until you get sick of them is a great approach to planning that is lighter on the mental load, because the meals become familiar (and therefore easier to make) and you can bulk shop for ingredients.

When your baby is in the clingy koala phase, their first nap of the day is a great time to cook in batches. Cook enough for lunch and dinner and pop the rest in the freezer. Do this a couple of times a week and you will end up with a wonderful selection of meals on rotation. Just remember to label them with what they are and date they were made, so you can keep track of what's in there and what needs eating. A marker and masking tape are excellent for this and can live in your kitchen drawer for easy access.

JUST HEAT IT

Some days you aren't going to feel like eating your boring old freezer meal, but the moment you heat it and the smell hits your nostrils, you usually remember how delicious your frozen meal is and why you made it in the first place. And if you just can't bear the thought of yet another bowl of that frozen minestrone, drop it on a friend's doorstep for them to heat and enjoy. This is the exact kind of community spirit that keeps the village alive.

CLICK AND COLLECT YOUR GROCERIES!

Not having to get your baby (or toddler) out of the car at the supermarket is game changing. It helps you save money because you make less impulse purchases when you're not in-store, and you can do it in the evening once your child/ren are asleep, making it easier to create and adhere to a shopping list. You might find having groceries delivered is an even bigger lifesaver, so you don't have to get in the car at all! Be sure to stock up on non-perishable items, including frozen greens, tinned beans, sardines, nuts, seeds and eggs, so that even when the fridge is bare you can whip up something nutritious.

FEEDING FUSSPOTS

If your kids have no interest in eating what you eat, feed them snack plates or deconstructed versions of your own meals. Remember to include a starchy carbohydrate, fruit or veg, protein and healthy fat with every meal, then trust they will get what they need. Unless your child has sensory aversions to certain foods, the consensus is that you should act unfazed if they refuse a food or go through a fussy phase, and eventually, it will pass. Feeding Littles is an excellent resource.

Hot Tip:

Keep a pen and notepad in your kitchen and write things on it as you run out of them. Bye-bye last minute supermarket runs when you are about to make dinner and realise you've forgotten x, y or z.

Household Chores

It's nice to get a bit of cooking or laundry done while they are napping, but if your child is still waking in the night, you need to rest during the day as well, period. Consider napping while they do, and involve them in the housework during waking hours. Put on some music and have a little boogie together while you tick off your to-do list. Kids LOVE the sense of agency and responsibility that comes with helping and it allows you to turn household chores into a fun game. Sometimes they make it impossible, yes, and sometimes you feel guilty for saying no to playing because you need to hang out the laundry first. But if you can use one of their naps to have a nap too (even if only on the weekends), you will be parenting from a more rested and resourced place, and will thus have more to give.

And on the days you get 'nothing' done – take stock. How are you measuring your worth? Is it by the number of dishes washed and clothes put away, or by the number of toddler tears turned into smiles?

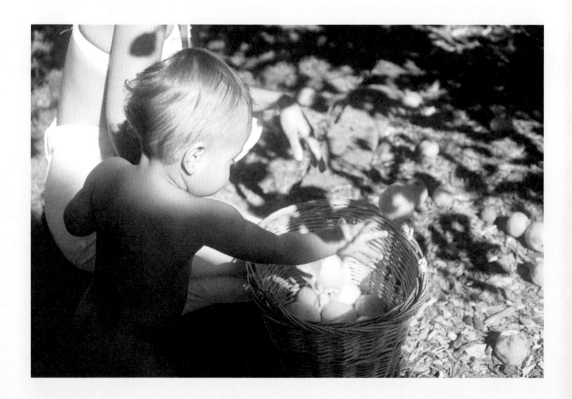

Returning to Work

Returning to work is a HUGE topic and, as with everything in parenthood, there is no one-size-fits-all scenario or approach. Whatever you decide is deeply personal. Regardless of whether you work for yourself or someone else, work can be fraught with anxiety and overwhelm, even if you love your job.

If you have a partner, it can be valuable to consider your working hours as a family unit. If you are both working full time with inflexible hours, it's going to be difficult to tend to the needs of your children while managing your home, caring for yourself and maintaining friendships.

Thankfully, society is changing, albeit slowly. More people are self-employed or abandoning the nine to five grind in favour of flexible working hours that allow a healthier work–life balance. Conscious professional coach Alison Rice advises 'it might help you to redefine what it means to "earn". In each chapter or season, we earn what's most relevant for us. Sometimes we earn money. Sometimes we earn time and flexibility. Sometimes we earn relationships, family and friends.'

Regardless of how it looks for you, being a working mother can be challenging and a lot of paid work isn't compatible with full-time parenthood. Sociologist and motherhood expert Dr Sophie Brock calls this the Care–Career Conundrum and reminds us that mothers will experience guilt because society is not set up to support mothers, especially not working mothers.

'Mothers are stuck between an economy that tells them the work comes first and a society that tells them the kids come first, but who is advocating for the mothers' needs? The result is an entire generation of burnt-out women.'

DAPHNE DELVAUX, ESQ.

MUM GUILT AND THE PERFECT MOTHER MYTH

BY DR SOPHIE BROCK

If all this talk of connection and play, and going back to work, and remaining calm through the storm of motherhood while making sure your kids are fed and have clean clothes that fit them, and, and, and ... has you riddled with guilt, you are not alone. In fact, for many, the guilt can manifest as anger or rage, as you buckle under the tremendous pressure of it all.

Dr Sophie Brock uses her Anger–Guilt Trap™ model to explain why 'The Perfect Mother Myth' leads to cycles of anger and guilt in motherhood.

How mothers experience motherhood is shaped by many factors, including the social and cultural context they live within. Society has set up a particular ideal of what it means to be a 'perfect mother', represented by 'The Perfect Mother Myth'. This myth sets up an unrealistic and idealised version of what it means to be a mother, including feeling nothing but blissful, grateful and happy, sacrificing her all for the sake of her children, and never putting herself first. There are many other parts of The Perfect Mother Myth that mean most mothers struggle to even begin to ever 'live up' to it. This leaves mothers feeling as though they are never good enough, and the internalisation of The Perfect Mother Myth through how we're socialised into motherhood means for most mothers, the experience is plagued by feelings of guilt.

This is explained through the Anger–Guilt Trap™ model where mothers try to make up for the guilt they experience through placing more pressure on themselves to self-sacrifice, to give more, to do more, to be more. In other words, to try and have themselves 'fit' more closely within the rules of The Perfect Mother Myth. This striving can contribute to and exacerbate depletion because of the cultural and social construct we're living in, where most mothers are inadequately supported. As mothers sacrifice more and it never seems to be enough, they can end up feeling resentful, like they're giving their all and are not valued. Eventually, a breaking point is met where the anger and resentment bubbling away can erupt to the surface. This expression of anger – especially because it is outside of The Perfect Mother Myth – leads to guilt. This is how the Anger–Guilt Trap™ continues as a cycle.

While anger and guilt are actually normal and can even be healthy parts of motherhood, when mothers feel like they are trapped in a cycle of anger and guilt that is fuelled by The Perfect Mother Myth, it can pervade the whole experience of being a mum.

Sophie shares some tips as to how we can use our anger and guilt as a vehicle for change:

1. Understand the Anger–Guilt Trap™ and start identifying when we're within it.
2. Get curious about what our guilt and anger are revealing to us.
3. Understand the social construction of motherhood and detox from The Perfect Mother Myth – get clear on YOUR values.
4. Embrace and expect maternal ambivalence – feeling two seemingly opposing feelings (i.e. I'm so fulfilled by mothering/I'm so bored by mothering) are not only normal but important for us and our children.
5. Foster self-connection practices and reach out for support. Connection helps to combat shame and this can change how we experience (and express) anger. This can create hugely positive ripple effects in our mothering.

The Anger-Guilt Trap™ in Motherhood

BY DR SOPHIE BROCK

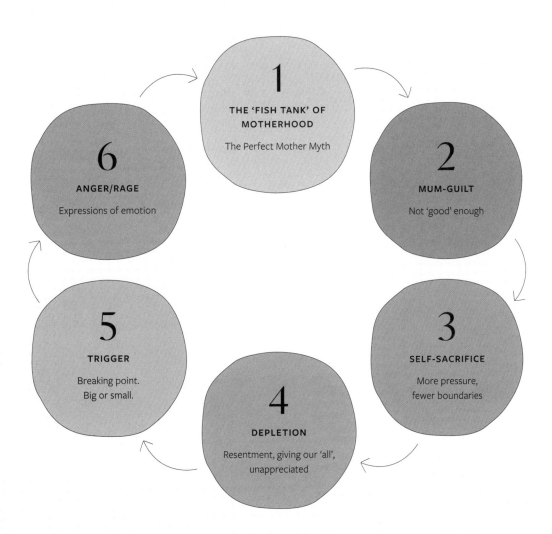

1

THE 'FISH TANK' OF MOTHERHOOD

The Perfect Mother Myth

2

MUM-GUILT

Not 'good' enough

3

SELF-SACRIFICE

More pressure, fewer boundaries

4

DEPLETION

Resentment, giving our 'all', unappreciated

5

TRIGGER

Breaking point. Big or small.

6

ANGER/RAGE

Expressions of emotion

Copyright Dr Sophie Brock 2022
Image has been reproduced by permission from the author.

Last But Not Least

If we could share only one tip about parenting it would be this: if something isn't working, change it.

You probably had a notion about how easily your child would fit into your schedule, how well they would sleep, eat, 'behave', etc., and how you would parent accordingly. We encourage you to let go of how you *thought* you would do things and come back to what we said at the beginning of this book – surrender.

Use your intuition to guide you towards what will work best for you and your family, and ignore what you think you 'should' be doing. Ask for help. Have honest and constructive conversations with those close to you so that you can put plans in place to help you and your family thrive. Remember – unless we are taking care of ourselves, we simply cannot give our children the best versions of ourselves.

It may take a while to find your groove and even when you do, things will be bumpy at times. Even though no two families are the same, as someone on the roller-coaster of parenthood, you are not alone. There will be days where you feel stretched beyond your wildest imagination, but even the worst days will be filled with more love than you ever knew possible. Such is the duality of motherhood.

Hang in there, you got this. It really is the longest shortest time.

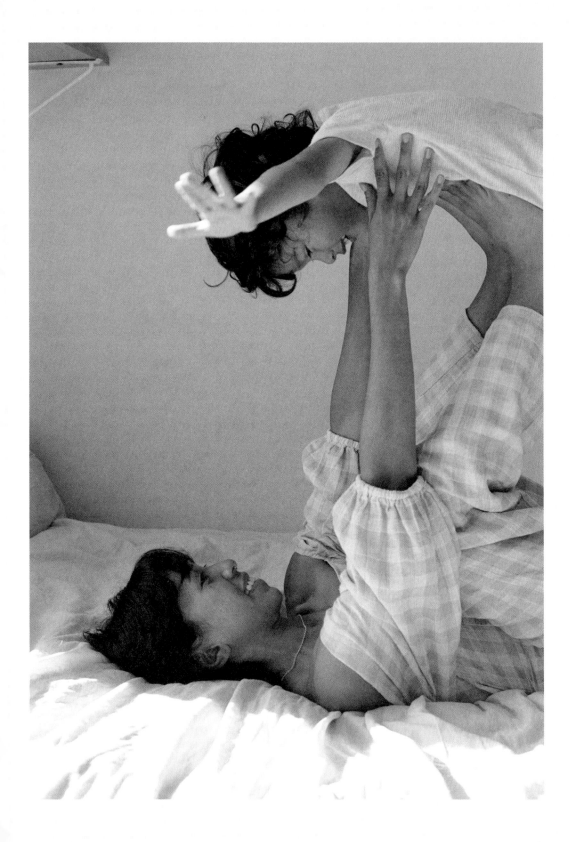

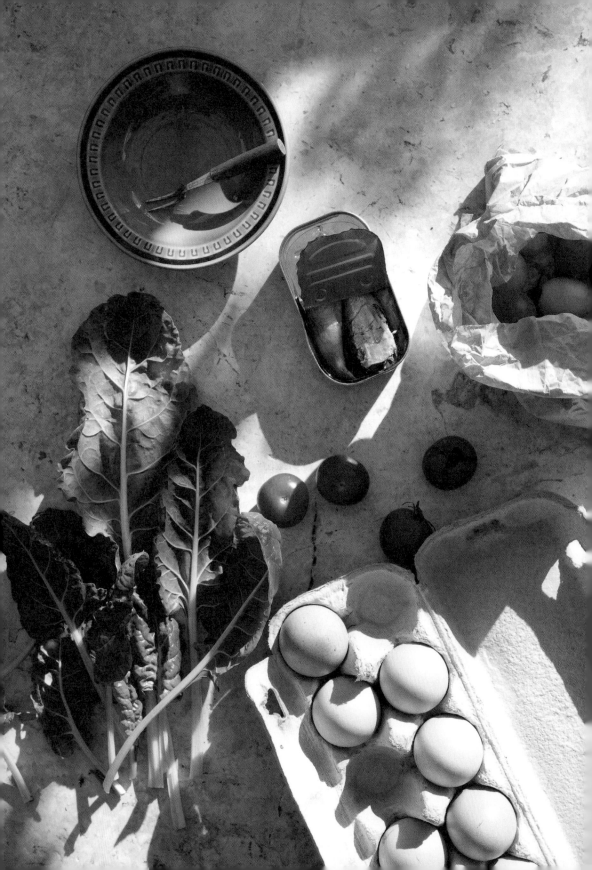

SIMPLE

CHAPTER SIX

RECIPES

We are obsessed with food.

We love cooking it, we love eating it, and we literally never stop talking about it. We love it so much that we started Mama Goodness together – a business that delivers food to new mums in Melbourne (where we live).

This is by no means a comprehensive postpartum recipe guide. We didn't have the space, and there are already so many incredible resources available with a focus on meals and nutrition for the first few weeks at home with your babe, so we wanted to share recipes that complement, rather than compete with what's out there.

On the following pages you will find simple yet deeply nourishing recipes that you can make not only in pregnancy and your immediate postpartum, but when you are a mother to toddlers, school kids and even teenagers. Most of the recipes contain options for both meat and plant proteins, and they are chock full of nature's greatest source of nutrients, antioxidants and fibre: plants.

No matter if you are vegan, vegetarian, pescatarian, flexitarian or omnivore, studies show that eating a predominantly plant-based diet is best for overall health. It is also recommended that we consume at least thirty different plant foods a week for optimal gut flora diversity, as gut health is linked to mood and immunity, as well as our ability to absorb nutrients from our food.

We are pretty passionate about encouraging our postpartum mamas and Mama Goodness customers to consume more plants, not only because of their innumerable health benefits, but also because a plant-heavy diet is a lot lighter on the planet than a meat-heavy one. In a time where the planet needs us to step up and make small changes that will have a big impact, our plates are a wonderful place to start.

The recipes in the pages that follow are environmentally friendly, simple to make, create minimal mess and will hopefully inspire you when you are in a food rut. They are accessible for beginner cooks and chefs alike, and most cook within an hour (many of them MUCH less). This is the type of food you can throw together with a baby on your hip, and that you can make in bulk and freeze to eat in the weeks and months to come.

As we said in the previous chapter – aim to cook more, less often. Lean into the simplicity of batch cooking the same meals, and as you get to know your favourites, you will be able to make them with ease, which is a blessing for the mental load.

There is a large focus on leafy greens, oats, eggs and legumes, because these foods provide the foundations for optimal nutrition in the postpartum. We recommend avoiding processed meats, and opting instead for grass-fed animal products that come from reputable sources such as local farms and organic butchers. The healthier the animals are and the less hormones or antibiotics they've received, the better their meat is for you.

Contents

Please note this book uses 20 ml (¾ fl oz) tablespoons. Cooks using 15 ml (½ fl oz) tablespoons should be mindful of slightly increasing the amount with their tablespoon measurements. Metric cup measurements are used, i.e. 250 ml (8½ fl oz) for 1 cup. In the US 1 cup is 8 fl oz (235 ml), so American cooks should be generous with their cup measurements; in the UK, a cup is 10 fl oz (295 ml), so British cooks should be scant. Additionally, the recipes in this book were cooked in a conventional oven. The general rule tells us that if using a fan-forced or convection oven to reduce the temperature by 20°C (70°F).

QUICKEST EASIEST LACTATION COOKIES

MAKES 15 COOKIES

160 g (5½ oz/½ cup) maple
    syrup
200 g (7 oz/¾ cup) natural
    peanut butter
90 g (3¼ oz/scant 1 cup)
    ground almonds
90 g (3¼ oz/scant 1 cup) quick
    oats
1½ teaspoons baking powder
30 g (1 oz/¼ cup) cacao
    powder
1 tablespoon hemp seeds
1 tablespoon chia seeds
1 tablespoon ground linseeds
    (flax seeds)
1 teaspoon vanilla extract
pinch of salt

There is a version of these in Jess' One-Pot book and they are such a hit amongst the mamas in our life, we just had to include them in this book too.

We don't use brewer's yeast in this recipe because the amount required in order for it to have galactagogue properties makes the cookies taste horrendous. Instead, we use the galactagogue properties of oats, almonds and peanut butter with an added boost of omegas from our signature seed trio to bring you a cookie that's quick, easy and delicious.

Preheat the oven to 180°C (350°F) and line a tray with baking paper.

Combine the maple syrup and peanut butter in a bowl. If necessary, heat gently to loosen. Add the remaining ingredients and mix to combine.

Roll the mixture into 15 balls and place on the lined baking tray. Flatten them with a fork or your palm to about 1 cm (½ in) thick and bake for 8–10 minutes, or until you can smell them.

Remove from the oven and allow to cool on a tray.

These cookies will keep in an airtight jar for at least a month.

Pictured on pages 180–181, from
left to right: Umami Tahini Slice;
Oaty, Fudgy, Chocolate Slice;
Quickest Easiest Lactation Cookies.

UMAMI TAHINI SLICE

MAKES 10–15 SLICES

90 g (3 oz/⅓ cup) unhulled tahini
or almond butter

115 g (4 oz/⅓ cup) raw local
honey or maple syrup

40 g (1½ oz/¼ cup) cacao butter

large pinch of sea salt

25 g (1 oz/1½ cups) puffed brown
rice

25 g (1 oz/1 cup) puffed quinoa

35 g (1¼ oz/¼ cup) goji berries

35 g (1¼ oz/¼ cup) cacao nibs

55 g (2 oz/⅓ cup) pepitas
(pumpkin seeds), toasted

55 g (2 oz/½ cup) chopped
walnuts, toasted

sesame seeds and sea salt flakes,
to garnish

This slice is packed full of hormone-loving fats in the form of nuts, seeds and butters, and is the perfect amount of sweet and salty for that umami hit. Whenever we make this for clients or gatherings, adults and children inhale it at lightning speed.

We absolutely adore this specific combination of ingredients, but as with most of our recipes you can substitute with whatever nuts, seeds or dried fruits are in your cupboard, e.g. almonds instead of walnuts, cranberries instead of goji berries.

A reminder that children under the age of one shouldn't be given honey, so if you are making this with curious little eaters in mind, opt for maple syrup (and make sure your nuts are finely chopped).

Line a 15 cm × 30 cm (6 in × 12 in) loaf (bar) tin with baking paper. The baking paper should come up over the sides of the tin so that you can use the paper to lift the slice out later.

Gently melt the tahini, honey, cacao butter and salt in a small pot on a low heat. Keep an eye on it, as it can go from melted to burnt in the bat of an eyelid.

Combine the remaining ingredients in a large mixing bowl. Pour the melted ingredients into the dry mixture and stir. Pour the combined mixture into the lined tin and press down firmly. Sprinkle with sesame seeds and salt flakes.

Place in the fridge for a few hours or overnight to set.

Remove from the tray by lifting the baking paper. Cut into slices and store in the fridge in an airtight container for up to a month.

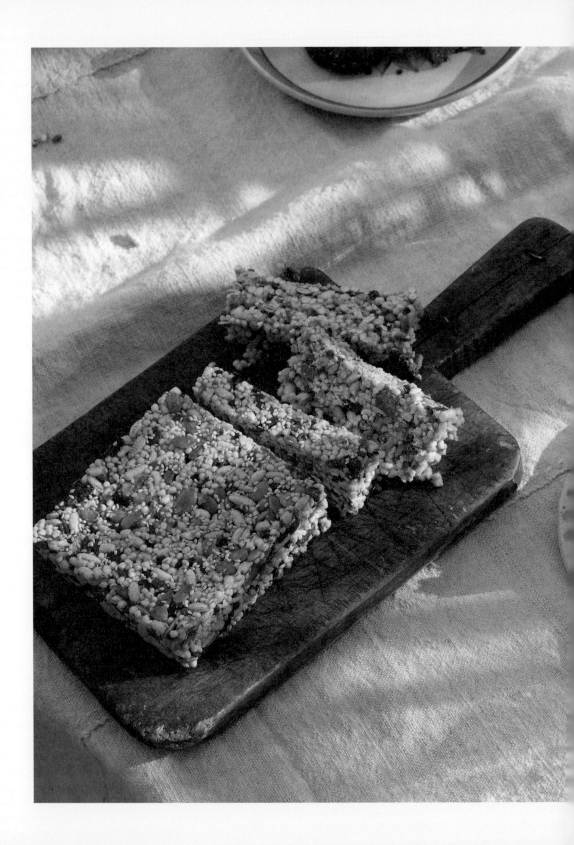

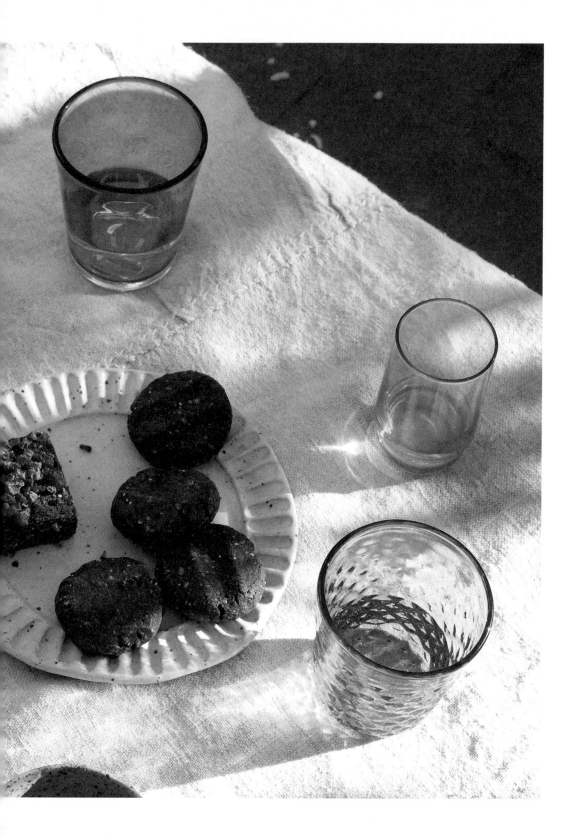

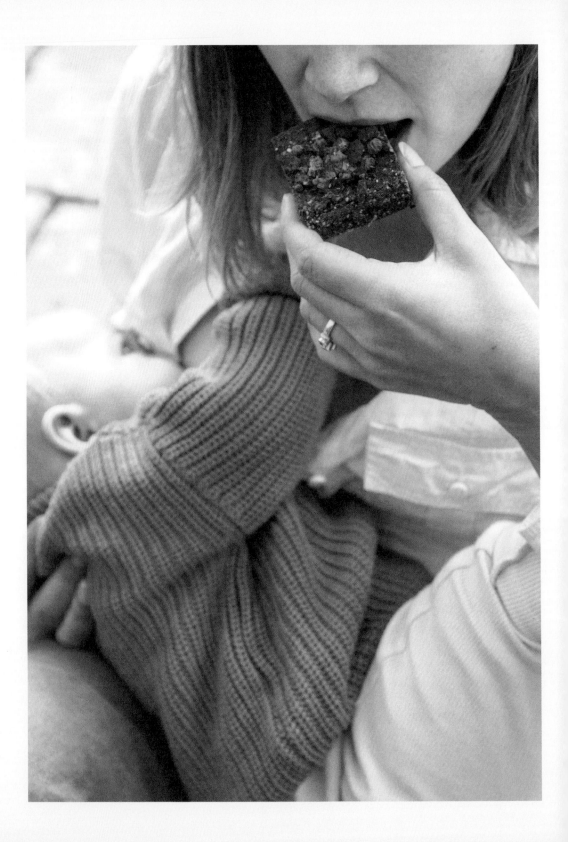

OATY, FUDGY, CHOCOLATE SLICE

MAKES 16–25 PIECES

10 fresh Medjool dates, pitted

120 g (4½ oz/¾ cup) sultanas
  (golden raisins)

90 g (3 oz/¾ cup) roasted almonds

70 g (2½ oz/½ cup) pepitas
  (pumpkin seeds)

40 g (1½ oz/¼ cup) hemp seeds

90 g (3 oz/1 cup) rolled (porridge)
  oats

90 g (3 oz/1 cup) desiccated
  (shredded) coconut

60 g (2 oz/½ cup) cacao powder

1 teaspoon vanilla

pinch of sea salt

280 g (10 oz/1 cup) natural peanut
  butter

120 g (4½ oz/½ cup) coconut oil,
  melted

freeze-dried raspberries, to garnish
  (optional)

Full of healthy fats and antioxidant-rich cacao powder, as well as the galactagogue goodness of oats and peanut butter – this slice really hits the spot.

Line a 20 cm × 20 cm (8 in x 8 in) tin with baking paper.

Place everything except the peanut butter and coconut oil in a food processor and pulse to a fine crumb (approximately 20 seconds). While the machine is running, add the peanut butter and coconut oil and process until combined.

Transfer the mixture into your baking tin and press firmly, using damp fingers or the back of a tablespoon. Once smooth and even, crush the freeze-dried raspberries over the top, if using. Place in the fridge for a few hours or overnight.

Remove from the tin by lifting the baking paper out. Cut into squares – 4 cm x 4 cm if you like a smaller slice, or 5 cm x 5 cm if you prefer a chunkier slice. You can also cut rectangles or triangles if you like – go wild!

Store in the fridge in an airtight container for up to a month.

CARROT AND BLUEBERRY BREAKFAST CAKES

MAKES 6–12 CAKES

coconut oil, for greasing

400 ml (13½ fl oz/1⅔ cups)
tinned coconut milk

2 tablespoons chia seeds

1 teaspoon apple-cider vinegar

230 g (8 oz/2 cups) grated
carrot (about 3 medium
carrots)

80 ml (2½ fl oz /⅓ cup) maple
syrup

80 ml (2½ fl oz/⅓ cup) olive
oil or melted coconut oil

200 g (7 oz/2 cups) quick oats

40 g (1½ oz/⅓ cup) goji berries

2 tablespoons hemp seeds

2 tablespoons ground linseeds
(flax seeds)

2 teaspoons ground ginger

1 teaspoon ground cinnamon

1 teaspoon vanilla extract

¼ teaspoon ground nutmeg

1 teaspoon bicarbonate of soda
(baking soda)

1 teaspoon baking powder

pinch of sea salt

50 g (1¾ oz/½ cup) walnuts

115 g (4 oz/¾ cup) fresh or
frozen blueberries

To serve:

coconut yoghurt

lemon zest

milk of your choice

The original recipe for these little cakes is from Jess' Vegan One-Pot Wonders cookbook, and it has a cult status amongst the mums in our community. We put it on our Mama Goodness menu, and the cult status only intensified, so we just had to include it in this book! We have added postpartum friendly goji berries, hemp seeds and linseeds, making it the perfect meal or snack for any time of day (or 'Breakfast, Lunch and Dinner Cake' as some of our postpartum clients call it).

Preheat the oven to 160°C (320°F) and grease the muffin tin (12-hole standard muffin tin or 6-hole giant muffin tin) with coconut oil.

Combine the coconut milk, chia seeds and apple-cider vinegar in a bowl and leave to curdle while you peel and grate the carrots.

Add the maple syrup, olive oil and grated carrot to the wet mixture, stir well then add all the dry ingredients and stir until well combined. Fold in the blueberries then pour the mixture into the muffin tin and place in the oven for 20–30 minutes, until golden on top and crisp around the edges.

Remove from oven and allow to sit for 10 minutes. Serve warm, topped with coconut yoghurt and lemon zest, or in a bowl with your milk of choice.

Store in the fridge for up to 4 days or freeze for up to 3 months.

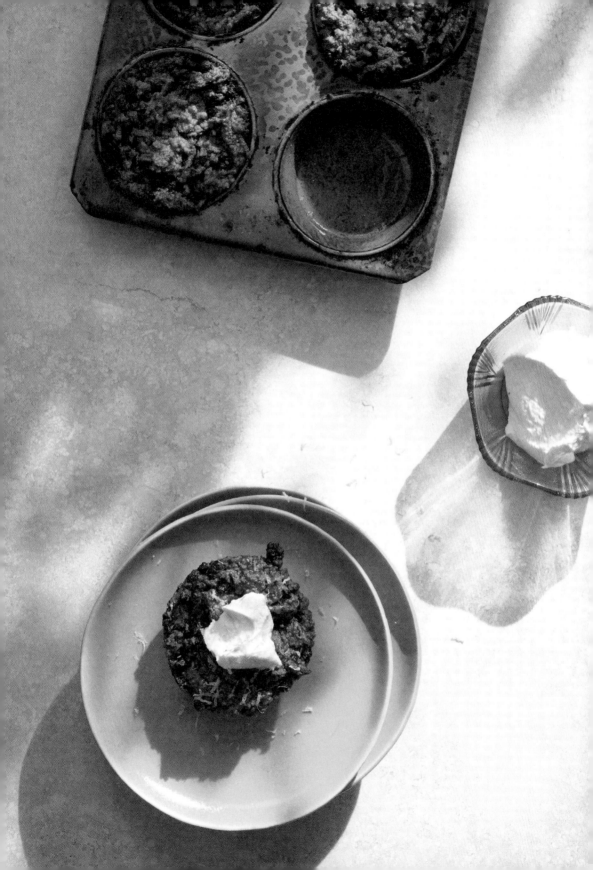

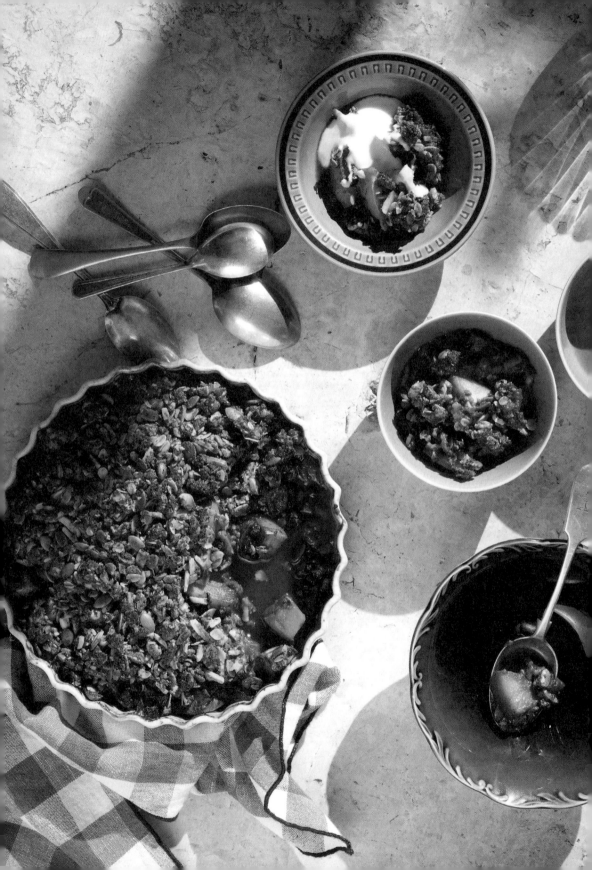

ANYTHING AND EVERYTHING CRUMBLE

SERVES 4

**For the fruit filling (aim to
have approx. 6 cups fruit
all up)**
2–3 apples, cut into 1.5 cm (½ in)
chunks
2–3 pears, cut into 1.5 cm (½ in)
chunks
125 g (4½ oz/1 cup) raspberries
155 g (5½ oz/1 cup) blueberries
juice of 1 lemon
1 teaspoon coconut sugar

For the crumble topping
50 g (1¾ oz/½ cup) rolled
(porridge) oats
60 g (2 oz/½ cup) oat flour
60 g (2 oz/½ cup) slivered
almonds
70 g (2½ oz/½ cup) pepitas
(pumpkin seeds)
85 g (3 oz/½ cup) coconut sugar
zest of 1 lemon
generous splash of vanilla
100 g (3½ oz) grass-fed butter
or coconut oil

To serve:
full-fat cream or yoghurt
of choice

*Who doesn't love a crumble? Jess has the fondest memories of her dear friend Nina
dropping a crumble on her doorstep after she had Jude. The simplest gestures really
do mean so much.*

*We've called this anything and everything crumble because – so long as you keep the
ratios the same – you can go wild with ingredients. Are we noticing a theme here?*

*We leave the skin on our fruit as it's an excellent source of nutrients and fibre, but you
can peel it too if you prefer the texture of skin-free fruit in your crumble.*

Preheat the oven to 180°C (360°F).

Place the fruit in a mixing bowl along with the lemon juice and sugar. Toss to combine,
then transfer to a pie dish and bake for 20–30 minutes until the fruit begins to soften,
stirring once during the cooking time.

Place all crumble ingredients in a mixing bowl and work the butter into the topping with
your fingertips. Once the fruit has started to soften, stir once more and then cover
with the topping and return to the oven for 40 minutes.

Allow to cool for 10 minutes, then serve with full fat cream, yoghurt or coconut yoghurt.

OATY GOODNESS

SERVES 7

4 tablespoons slivered almonds

4 tablespoons sunflower kernels

4 tablespoons pepitas (pumpkin seeds)

2 tablespoons hemp seeds

2 tablespoons chia seeds

2 tablespoons ground linseeds (flax seeds)

2 tablespoons goji berries

350 g (12½ oz/3½ cups) rolled (porridge) oats

1 teaspoon vanilla powder

By now you've probably cottoned on to the power of oats in the postpartum. They are full of fibre, iron and are one of the best known galactagogues. Delicious and nutritious as they are, as a naturopath, Vaughne doesn't recommend eating them on their own, as doing so will cause a spike in your blood sugar levels and cause you to feel hungry not long after eating them. Instead, she recommends pairing them with protein, which will ensure they keep you fuller for longer.

This dry mix is packed full of protein and fibre, making it the perfect thing for you to prepare when you're pregnant. You can then use it to make either porridge or overnight oats, depending on what time of year it is and what your body is craving. Genius, right?

Preheat the oven to 200°C (390°F). Scatter the almonds, sunflower kernels and pepitas on a baking tray and toast in the oven for 5 minutes. Leave to cool.

In a large bowl, combine the toasted mixture with the remaining ingredients and stir to combine. Transfer to an airtight jar.

To make overnight oats:
Place 75 g (¾ cup) Oaty Goodness with 375 ml (12½ fl oz/1½ cups) milk of your choice in a bowl.

Sweeten with a tablespoon of maple syrup if you like, or a splash of vanilla extract if you were unable to add vanilla powder to your dry mix.

Pop in the fridge overnight. In the morning, give it a good stir and top with a dollop of nut butter or yoghurt and our Spiced Digestive Compote (overleaf) or fresh fruit of your choice.

To make porridge:
Place 75 g (¾ cup) Oaty Goodness with 375 ml (12½ fl oz/1½ cups) milk of your choice in a small saucepan over a medium heat. Cook, stirring often, for about 5 minutes, or until oats are thick and creamy.

Sweeten with a tablespoon of maple syrup if you like, or a splash of vanilla extract if you were unable to add vanilla powder to your dry mix.

Transfer to a bowl and top with a dollop of nut butter or yoghurt and our Spiced Digestive Compote (overleaf) or fresh fruit of your choice.

The best of both worlds:
Soak Oaty Goodness mixture overnight then heat, top and eat in the morning for the ultimate, creamiest porridge.

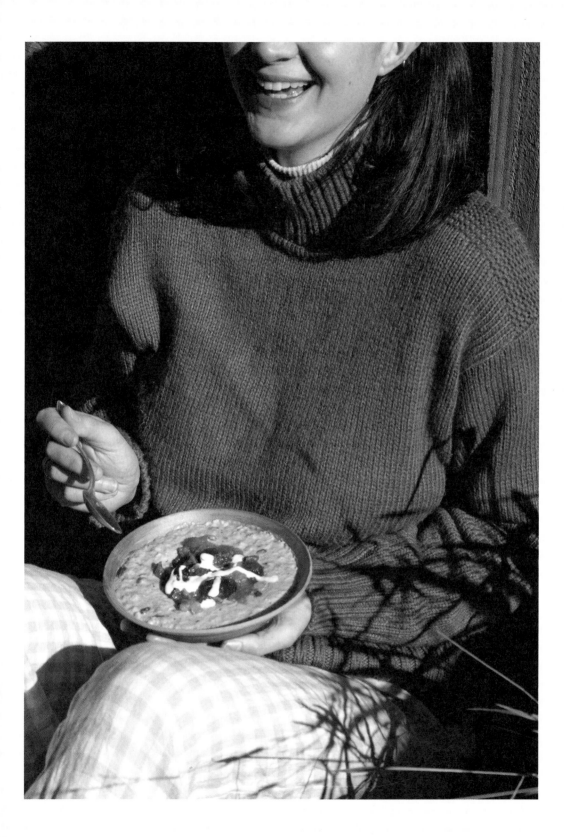

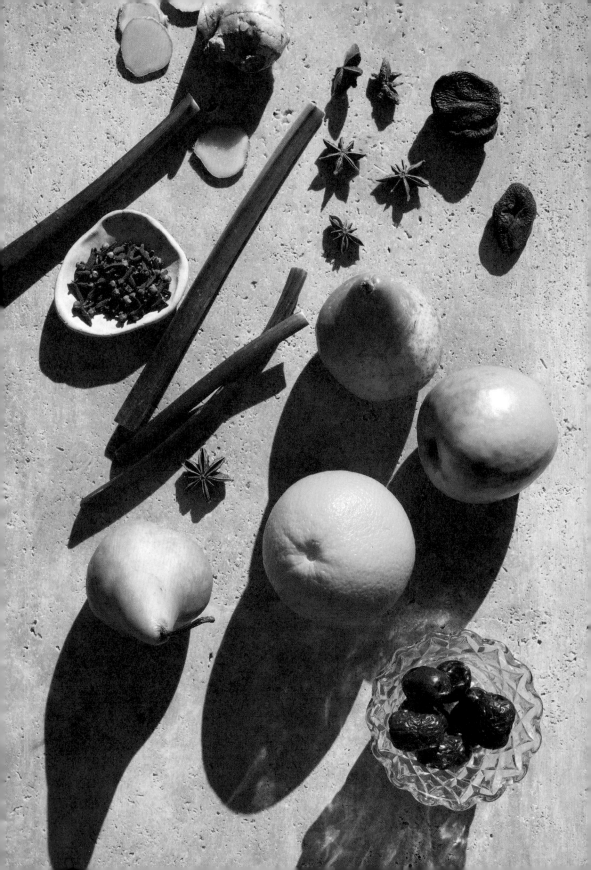

SPICED DIGESTIVE COMPOTE

SERVES 4–8

3 granny smith apples, peeled
  and chopped into 3 cm
  (1¼ in) chunks

3 pears, peeled and chopped
  into 3 cm (1¼ in) chunks

6–8 stalks rhubarb, leaves
  removed, stalks cut into 3 cm
  (1¼ in) pieces

200 g (7 oz/approx. 18) prunes,
  halved and stones removed

100 g (3½ oz/approx. 16) dried
  apricots, halved

50 g (1¾ oz/approx. 16) Chinese
  red dates

thumb-sized piece of ginger,
  peeled and sliced

2 cinnamon sticks

2 star anise

1 orange, juiced, rind peeled into
  thick ribbons

a few cloves, pushed into the
  orange rind

If there's a recipe that your guts will love, this is it! When you need a little help getting things moving, this juicy, aromatic compote uses warming spices and fibre-rich fruit and vegetables to support your digestive system and help keep you regular.

This is great to eat right after you've had your baby, to help with your first postpartum poo. It's also great for constipated little ones. Just be sure to remove the whole spices as they could be a choking hazard.

Place the fruit and spices in a large saucepan. Add the orange juice, rind and 500 ml (17 fl oz/2 cups) water, and stir. The fruit won't be fully covered but as everything cooks and reduces, it will slowly become submerged in its own juices.

Cook on high until boiling. Reduce heat and simmer for 10–15 minutes, stirring occasionally. Press the pieces of fruit at the top down into the bubbling goodness.

Turn off the heat and leave for 10–15 minutes. The mixture will continue to soften as it cools.

Once cool, transfer to a glass container. Keeps in the fridge for up to 2 weeks and freezes beautifully. Use on top of your porridge or Oaty Goodness, or top with yoghurt and nuts.

Tip: If rhubarb is not in season, add an extra apple and pear to substitute.

LITTLE LOAF OF GOODNESS

MAKES 10–15 SLICES

190 g (6½ oz) rolled (porridge)
    oats
180 g (6½ oz) almonds
100 g (3½ oz) walnuts
80 g (2¾ oz) pepitas (pumpkin
    seeds)
40 g (1½ oz) hemp seeds
40 g (1½ oz) ground linseeds
    (flax seeds)
40 g (1½ oz) chia seeds
50 g (1¾ oz/4 tablespoons)
    psyllium husk
1½ teaspoons salt
3 tablespoons olive oil
1 tablespoon maple syrup

The idea for this slice came from none other than Sarah Britton of My New Roots, who has since inspired countless spins on this wheat-free and fibre-filled loaf. In our version, we've included our beloved hemp, chia and linseed trio, as well as pepitas and a whole lotta almonds.

The oats and psyllium husk make it the perfect first food after labour. Enjoy on its own – toasted and smeared with butter – or load it with hummus, tomato and avocado for something more substantial. The oats are a galactagogue, meaning they will support breastmilk production, and psyllium husk will help keep your digestion moving which, as discussed in chapter three, is important for that first postpartum poo!

Line a 10 cm × 20 cm (4 in x 8 in) loaf (bar) tin with baking paper.

Combine the dry ingredients in a large mixing bowl. Add the olive oil and maple syrup, along with 500 ml (17 fl oz/2 cups) water and stir until well combined. Transfer to the lined tin and firmly press into the tin, smoothing the top with the back of a tablespoon. Place in the fridge overnight.

The next day, preheat the oven to 200°C (390°F).

Place the loaf tin in the hot oven and bake for 30 minutes. Remove from the oven, lift the loaf out of the tin, remove the paper and place the loaf back in the oven – upside down and directly on the baking rack.

Bake for a further 30–40 minutes. Once cooked, it should sound hollow when you tap it.

Allow to cool, then slice.

Even though this loaf has been cooked, we recommend toasting each slice before eating, as doing so brings out the beautiful flavours of all those delicious nuts and seeds.

Store in an airtight container for up to a week. This loaf also freezes beautifully, just be sure to slice it first.

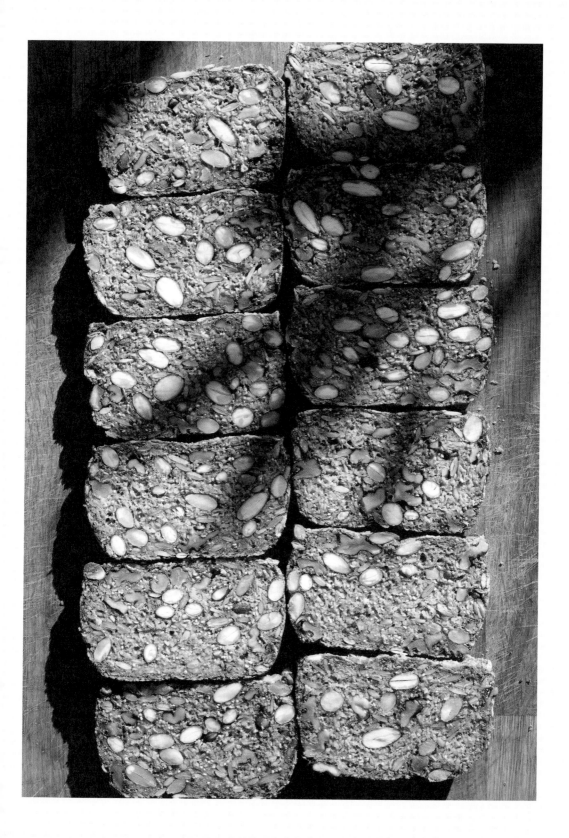

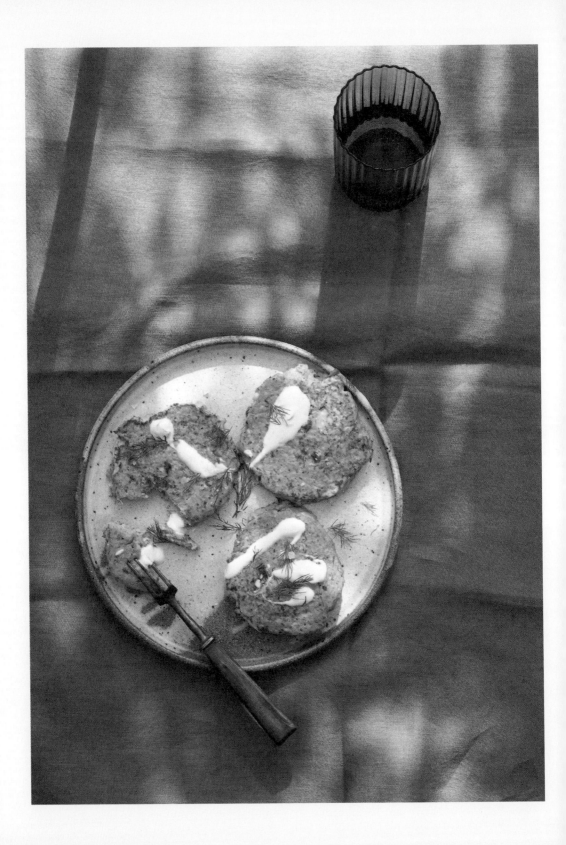

SWEET POTATO SALMON CAKES

MAKES 15 PALM-SIZED PATTIES

1 medium sweet potato (500 g/ 1 lb 2 oz), cut into chunks and boiled until soft

500 g (1 lb 2 oz) tinned wild caught salmon, with bones, drained and mashed

3 eggs

25 g (1 oz/¼ cup) ground almonds

2 tablespoons fresh dill or herbs of your choice (we love coriander/cilantro and flat-leaf/Italian parsley)

3 spring onions (scallions, approx. 30 g/1 oz), thinly sliced

1 tablespoon lemon zest

1 teaspoon sea salt

olive oil or ghee for cooking

To serve:

lemon juice

tzatziki

herbs to garnish

When it comes to adding brain-boosting and hormone-loving fats to your plate during the postpartum, these fish cakes are the business. You can swap salmon with other sustainably caught fish, such as mackerel or sardines if you have some in your pantry. This is one of the easiest, most palatable and nutrient dense ways to enjoy fish, as they are jam packed with DHA, with the addition of calcium when bones are left in, fibre from sweet potato and an added boost of protein from eggs and ground almonds. These freeze beautifully and are perfect to prepare during your pregnancy to pull out on days as a new mama when you need fuel but don't have the time or energy to cook.

Combine all ingredients in a large bowl and mash all ingredients together using a fork. Season with pepper to taste. Form the salmon mix into palm-sized patties.

Heat 1 tablespoon of olive oil or ghee in a frying pan over a medium–high heat. Cook the patties in batches, cooking on one side for 3 minutes and gently flipping before cooking on the other side for a further 3 minutes. Repeat with remaining patties.

Enjoy with a squeeze of lemon juice and drizzle of tzatziki.

Store in the fridge for up to 4 days. Leftovers can be frozen for up to 4 weeks. These can be defrosted and warmed in a low to medium pan with some ghee or in the microwave.

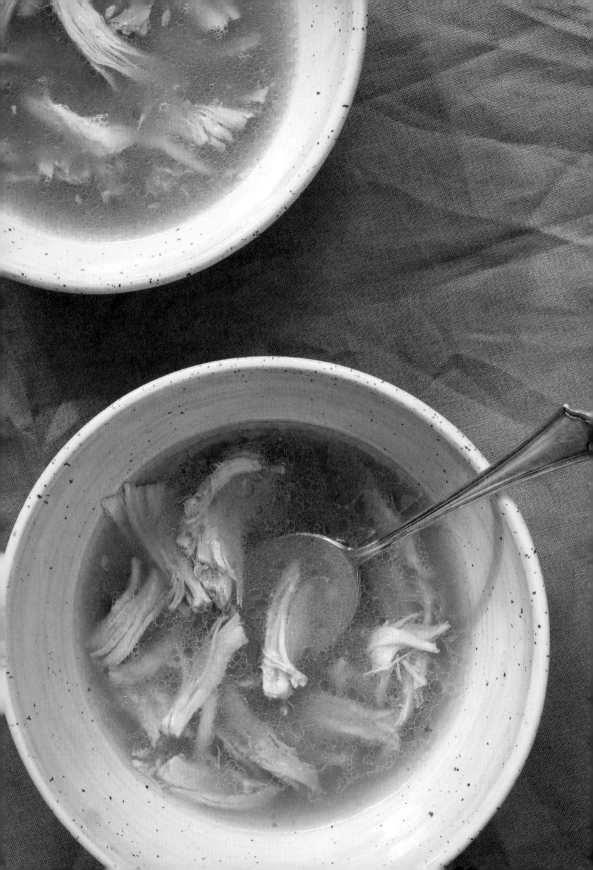

BROTH BROTH BABY

**MAKES 2.5 LITRES
(85 FL OZ/10 CUPS)**

1 whole organic chicken
2 carrots, roughly chopped
2 celery stalks, roughly chopped
1 medium onion, halved and
    peeled
4 garlic cloves
50 g (1¾oz) or thumb-sized
    piece of ginger, roughly
    chopped
1 cinnamon stick
2 bay leaves
1 teaspoon black peppercorns
¼ teaspoon cayenne pepper
filtered water, approx. 3 litres
    (101 fl oz/12 cups) (you can
    boil your kettle then allow
    to cool)

This recipe is so easy you could do it with your eyes half closed, which we know is how many mamas are cooking in the early postpartum. The beauty of this broth is that it uses the whole chicken, so you are left with plenty of poached meat which can be used for lunch or dinner in the days that follow.

This broth is rich in collagen, vitamins and minerals, as well as the amino acids glycine and arginine which are anti-inflammatory and support hormone health as well as skin, muscle and joint recovery.

Place the whole chicken, followed by all other ingredients in a large heavy-based stock pot and cover with the filtered water to approximately 5 cm (2 in) above the chicken.

Bring to the boil and then cover and reduce heat to low, allowing to simmer for 5 to 6 hours until the chicken is falling off the bone.

Remove from the heat and carefully remove the chicken from the pot using tongs or forks. Separate the meat from the bones. Discard the bones and store the meat in the fridge for up to 4 days.

Using a metal colander, strain the liquid into a large mixing bowl, allow to cool slightly, then ladle the broth into glass bottles or jars. Serve hot, alone or with reserved chicken meat.

The broth can be stored in the fridge for 2 days or frozen for up to 3 months.

NB: If freezing, don't fill your container all the way to the top as the broth will expand as it's freezing and will crack the glass if it has nowhere to go.

MAGICAL HEALING BROTH

**MAKES APPROXIMATELY
3 LITRES (101 FL OZ/
12 CUPS)**

1 onion, skin on, quartered

1 carrot, roughly chopped

1 celery stalk, leaves and all,
   roughly chopped

50 g (1¾ oz) or thumb-sized
   piece of fresh ginger, sliced

6 to 8 garlic cloves, peeled

10 g (¼ oz) dried seaweed
   (wakame or kelp)

5 to 6 dried shiitake mushrooms
   (about 10 g/¼ oz)

5 or 6 Chinese red (jujube) dates

1 tablespoon goji berries

1 lemongrass stalk, halved
   lengthways

1 cinnamon stick

3 star anise

1 tablespoon coriander seeds

1 tablespoon white peppercorns

1½ teaspoons salt

1 teaspoon miso paste, to serve

*This broth is full of warming, healing and immune-boosting foods that provide
maximum nutrition in an easy-to-digest liquid. It's light enough that it can be sipped
from a mug, so you get all the goodness even when you don't have the appetite
for a full meal. Make it more substantial by serving with noodles and veggies a la
our Five Minute Noodle recipe on page 209.*

Place all the ingredients in a large pot, cover with 4 litres (135 fl oz/16 cups) water
and bring to the boil. Reduce the heat and simmer, covered, for 2 hours.

Remove from the heat and once cooled, strain through a sieve into another large pot
or bowl, then ladle the broth into jars.

To serve, place a teaspoon of miso paste in a mug. Add a small amount of warm broth,
stir until the miso paste is dissolved and then top up the mug with more broth.

Store the remaining broth in a glass jug in the fridge for up to a week, or freeze for
up to 3 months.

NB: If freezing, don't fill your container all the way to the top as the broth will expand
as it's freezing and will crack the glass if it has nowhere to go.

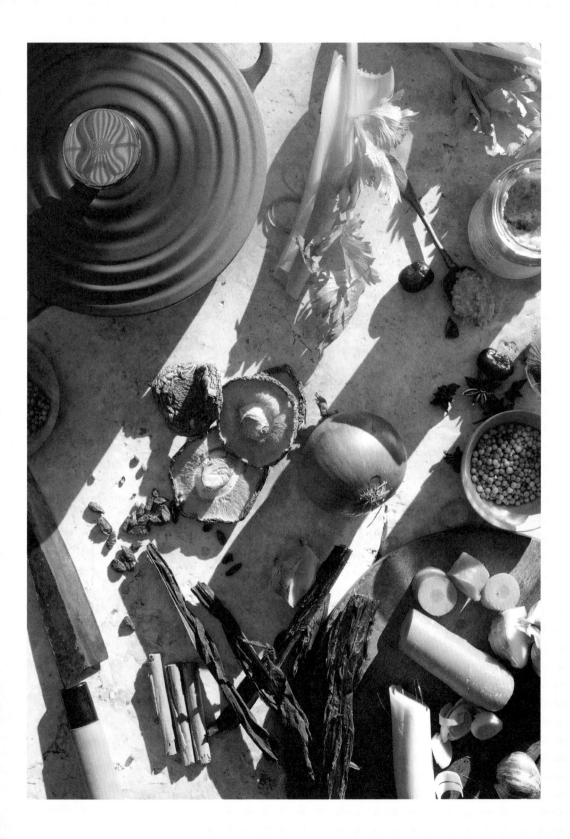

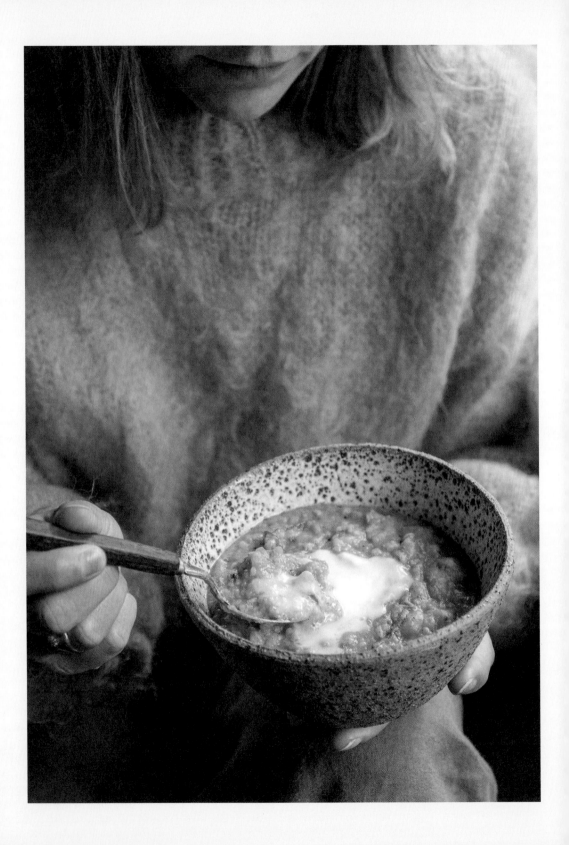

GOLDEN DAAL

SERVES 4–6

For the spice mix:
1 heaped tablespoon cumin
  seeds
1 heaped tablespoon ground
  coriander
1 heaped tablespoon ground
  turmeric
1 heaped tablespoon fennel
  seeds
1 teaspoon yellow mustard seeds
1 teaspoon ground fenugreek
½ teaspoon freshly ground black
  pepper
½ teaspoon asafoetida (hing
  powder)
½ teaspoon ground cinnamon
1 sprig curry leaves

For the daal:
4 tablespoons coconut oil
  or ghee
1 onion, diced
30 g (1 oz) fresh ginger, peeled,
  minced
3 garlic cloves, minced
2 teaspoons sea salt
200 g (7 oz) dried mung daal,
  rinsed or soaked overnight
  and drained
550 g (1 lb 3 oz) sweet potato,
  diced into 1 cm (½ in) cubes

To serve:
steamed basmati rice, or
  Indian flatbread,
unsweetened natural or
  coconut yoghurt (optional)
Indian chutney (optional)

There's nothing like a bowl of warming daal to make you feel nurtured and embraced. In our opinion, daal is one of the fundamental meals for postpartum. It's like a warm hug from an old friend, and the combination of gentle mung beans and therapeutic spices make it super supportive for even the most sensitive digestive system.

Combine the spices in a small bowl.

Warm 2 tablespoons of the coconut oil in a large saucepan over a medium–high heat.

Add the onion and ginger and cook for about 5 minutes, until the onion is starting to brown, then add the garlic and salt and cook for a minute before adding the drained daal, then fry for another minute.

Add the sweet potato and 1 litre (34 fl oz/4 cups) water, stir, cover and bring to the boil. Reduce the heat to low and simmer for 30 minutes, stirring every so often. Add an additional cup of water at the end of cooking time, if necessary, to achieve your desired consistency.

Heat the remaining oil in a large frying pan. Add the curry leaves and spices and cook for about a minute, stirring frequently, until leaves are fragrant and crispy, and the spices are starting to pop.

Pour the spice mix over the daal and stir to combine.

Ladle the daal into bowls and serve with basmati rice or Indian flatbread. Top with yoghurt and a spoonful of Indian chutney, if using.

Any leftovers will keep well in the fridge for a couple of days and it freezes beautifully. You may need to add water when reheating as it will thicken significantly when it cools.

Tip: You can soak uncooked basmati rice with the mung daal and add in at the same time, along with an extra teaspoon of salt and an extra litre of water. Voila, you've made kitchari, a warming Ayurvedic dish that is a popular postpartum meal.

MAMA GOODNESS SUPERGREEN LENTIL SOUP

SERVES 4–6

3 tablespoons olive oil

1 onion, finely chopped

3 carrots, diced

3 celery stalks, finely chopped

3 large or 5 small garlic cloves,
  finely chopped

2 tablespoons cumin seeds

1 teaspoon ground fenugreek

370 g (13 oz) black beluga lentils,
  soaked overnight

1 litre (34 fl oz/4 cups) stock/
  broth

250 g (9 oz) frozen greens
  (we use kale)

To serve:

squeeze of fresh lemon juice

toasted sourdough (optional)

Little Loaf of Goodness (p. 192,
  optional)

This soup has been on the Mama Goodness menu since we first launched in 2019. It is universally adored by kids and adults alike and we often receive messages from happy parents, thanking us for getting their kids to eat some greens. As with any soup, the key to getting the best flavour is using the best quality stock available to you, or even homemade chicken broth if you have any. We use frozen greens in this soup because they bring all the nutrition with none of the necessary washing and chopping, but you can absolutely use fresh leafy greens (our ultimate fave) if you have the time and energy to do so.

Heat the oil in a large saucepan over a medium heat, add the onion and cook for a couple of minutes until softened but not browned, then add the carrot and celery and cook for another 5–10 minutes until softened and starting to brown.

Add the garlic, cumin seeds and fenugreek and cook for about 2 minutes until fragrant.

Drain the lentils and add them to the pan along with the stock and 500 ml (17 fl oz/ 2 cups) water. Bring to the boil and cook for 20 minutes, or until the lentils squish easily on the side of the pan when pressed with a wooden spoon.

Once the lentils are cooked, add the greens and cook for another 5–10 minutes, then remove from the heat. Season to taste with salt and freshly ground black pepper.

Serve with a squeeze of fresh lemon juice, either alone or with a piece of toasted sourdough bread, or with our Little Loaf of Goodness (page 192).

The soup will keep for up to 5 days in an airtight container in the fridge, or in the freezer for up to 3 months.

Pictured on pages 204–205,
from bottom left to right:
Pumpkin and Coconut Stew,
Roasted Cauliflower Soup,
Mama Goodness Supergreen
Lentil Soup.

PUMPKIN AND COCONUT STEW

SERVES 4–6

3 tablespoons coconut oil
   or ghee
1 onion, diced
50 g (1¾ oz) fresh ginger,
   peeled, cut into matchsticks
3–4 garlic cloves, finely minced
4 makrut leaves, thinly sliced
1 kg (2 lb 3 oz) kent pumpkin,
   peeled and cut into bite-sized
   chunks
400 ml (3½ fl oz) tinned
   coconut milk
400 ml (13½ fl oz) vegetable
   stock or chicken broth
250 g (9 oz) tempeh, crumbled
1–2 bunches bok choy (pak
   choy), washed and chopped
   into bite-sized pieces

To serve:
cooked quinoa or rice
natural or plain coconut yoghurt
coriander leaves

If you've never tried tempeh, this recipe is a great place to start. It's made from fermented soybeans, and is an excellent source of lean protein while also being a fermented food containing prebiotics, which help to keep your gut flora healthy. If you're still not convinced, you can sub the tempeh for tofu, chicken, fish or beef and this stew will be just as delicious.

Heat the coconut oil in a large saucepan over a medium–high heat. Add the onion and ginger and cook for about 5 minutes, until the onion is translucent and ever so slightly starting to brown.

Add the garlic and makrut leaves and stir constantly for 1–2 minutes until fragrant, then add the pumpkin and stir to coat for 1 minute.

Add the coconut milk, stock and tempeh. Bring to a boil, then reduce the heat and simmer, covered, for 20 minutes, stirring occasionally. Once the pumpkin is tender enough that its edges are melding into the stew, add the greens, stirring to wilt and allow to cook for 3 minutes (longer if using frozen).

Taste and season with salt or pepper, if necessary (the stock might make it salty enough to not need additional seasoning).

Serve immediately with cooked quinoa or rice, topped with yoghurt and coriander leaves.

Any leftovers will keep well in the fridge for up to 4 days.

NB: The photo for this recipe (overleaf) doesn't contain greens, but there are meant to be greens in it, oops! Make it with or without, both ways are delicious.

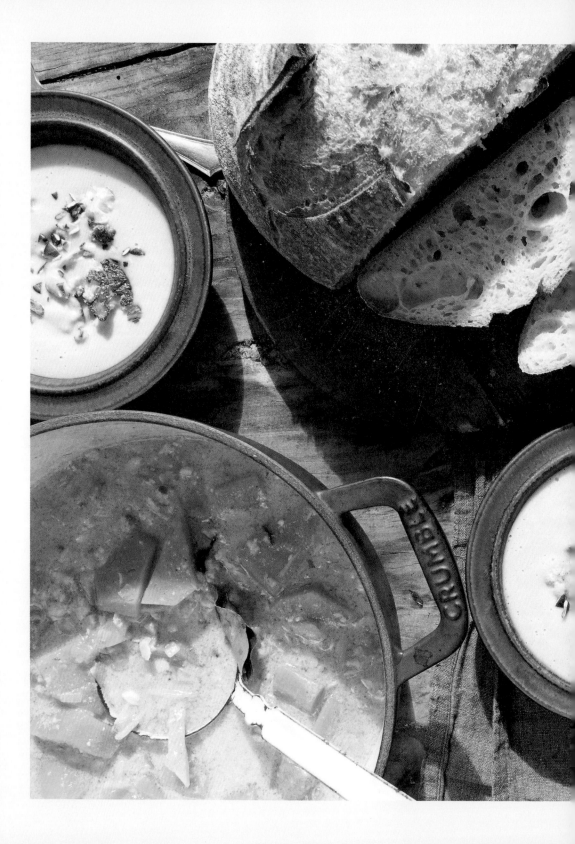

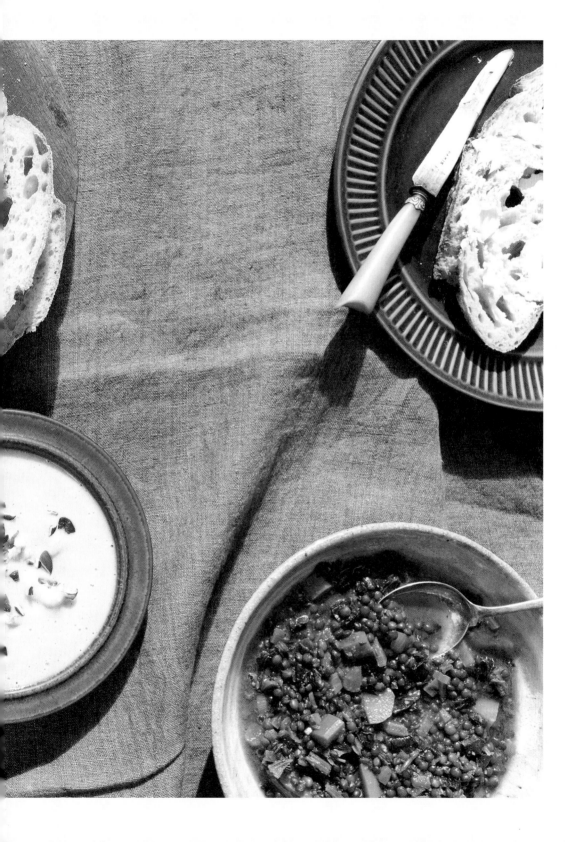

ROASTED CAULIFLOWER SOUP

SERVES 4–6

1 large (900 g/2 lb) cauliflower,
    cut into bite-sized florets
1 medium onion, peeled and cut
    into eighths
4 garlic cloves (skins intact)
½ teaspoon sea salt
1 teaspoon ground cumin
2–3 tablespoons olive oil
400 g (14 oz) tinned cannellini
    beans, drained and rinsed
1 litre (34 fl oz/4 cups) chicken
    broth or veggie stock
toasted pepitas (pumpkin
    seeds), to garnish
toasted sourdough bread,
    to serve

This creamy, dreamy, delicious soup is a bit of a sneaky recipe, because you don't actually make it in a pot! Instead, you roast the veggies, then blitz them in a blender with a can of beans and some hearty broth or stock.

Cauliflower is a cruciferous vegetable, which supports your liver and hormone health, while cannellini beans add creaminess with a boost of protein and fibre. We make this for all of our postpartum clients, and they gobble it up.

Preheat the oven to 220°C (430°F).

Place the cauliflower in a large mixing bowl, along with the onion and garlic. Add the salt, cumin and a generous glug of olive oil, and toss until the cauliflower is coated with the spice and oil mix.

Transfer to a baking tray and place in the oven for 30 minutes, tossing halfway through to ensure everything is evenly roasted. Allow to cool for 10 minutes.

In a blender, place half the cooked cauliflower, all the onion and all the garlic (remove skins first), along with the beans and cooled broth.

Purée on high until smooth, then stir in the remaining cauliflower. Add salt to taste.

Top with toasted pepitas and serve with toasted sourdough.

Tip: This dish is also outrageously good served with cooked pasta.

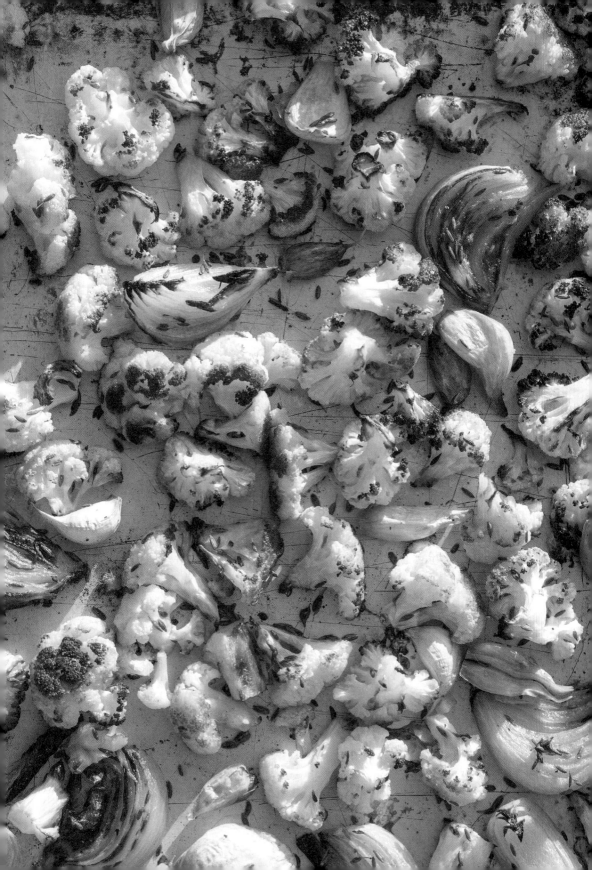

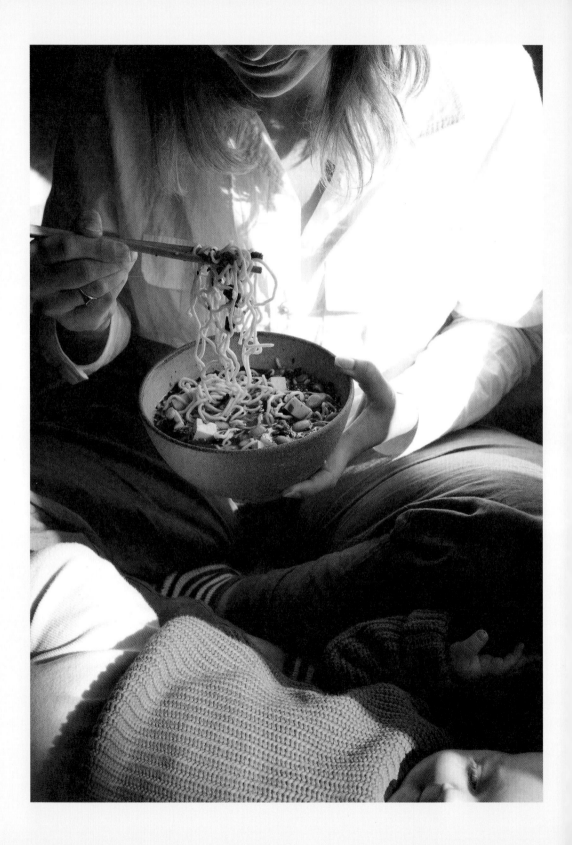

FIVE MINUTE NOODLES

SERVES 1

300 ml (10 fl oz) vegetable
    stock, Broth Broth Baby
    (p. 197) or Magical Healing
    Broth (p. 198)
125 g (4½ oz) soft tofu, cubed
100 g (3½ oz) dried noodles
50 g (1¾ oz) frozen edamame
70 g (2½ oz) frozen spinach
1 spring onion (scallion),
    chopped (optional)
1 teaspoon fresh ginger, grated
    (optional)
1 tablespoon toasted black
    and white sesame seeds,
    to garnish
tamari, to taste
sambal oelek (or other chilli
    sauce), to taste (optional)

You can throw these noodles together for a quick and easy meal on days when you're parenting solo. We always have these ingredients on hand, so even when we have 'nothing in the fridge' we can call on our trusty freezer and pantry and create this nourishing comfort meal in moments.

Bring the stock to a boil. Add the tofu and noodles and cook for 2 minutes.

Add the edamame, spinach, spring onion and ginger, if using. Stir frequently for about 3 minutes until the spinach has thawed and the noodles, beans and tofu are cooked.

Add a tablespoon of sesame seeds. Pour into a big bellied bowl and add tamari and sambal oelek (or other chilli sauce) to taste. Allow to cool for 5–10 minutes while you tend to other tasks, and then slurp your way to heaven.

NB: This recipe is based on noodles that take 5 minutes to cook. Check the packet to see if yours take longer, in which case cook them a little longer before adding the other ingredients.

Tips: You can substitute the tofu for 125 g cooked chicken, shredded.

Instead of noodles you can use 100 g spiralised zucchini.

GINGER RICE

SERVES 4–6

3 tablespoons toasted sesame
    oil
60 g (2 oz) fresh ginger, peeled,
    finely minced
6–8 garlic cloves, finely minced
400 g (14 oz/2 cups) jasmine rice
300–400 g (10½–14 oz) firm
    tofu, drained, pressed and cut
    into 1 cm (½ in) cubes
1 litre (34 fl oz/4 cups) vegetable
    stock, or chicken broth
300 g (10½ oz) frozen spinach
140 g (5 oz) frozen peas

Condiments

tamari or soy sauce
sambal oelek
Sesame Seaweed Sprinkles
    (p. 229)

To serve (optional):

soft boiled or fried egg
drizzle of toasted sesame oil
kimchi
toasted sesame seeds (if not
    using Sesame Seaweed
    Sprinkles)
ripe avocado, diced
chilli oil or sriracha (if not using
    sambal oelek)

A version of this was in Jess' One-Pot book and has since gained cult status in our community, where it is a firm favourite amongst friends, toddlers and doulas alike. In this version we use frozen spinach to make it even quicker and easier to prepare, and we've added frozen peas to bring even more green goodness with every bite. This is one of those recipes that you can make using the staples in your freezer and can be eaten as is, or topped with an egg.

Heat the sesame oil in a large saucepan over a medium heat. Add the ginger and garlic and cook for about 2 minutes until fragrant.

Add the rice and cook, stirring constantly for a couple of minutes, then add the tofu and stock. Cover, bring to the boil then lower the heat and simmer for 15 minutes.

Add the spinach and peas to the pot and stir into the rice to thaw more quickly. Cook for a further 2 minutes. Remove from the heat, stir, then cover and allow to sit for another 10 minutes while you gather the condiments and dice the avocado (if using).

Spoon the rice into bowls and serve with your favourite condiments and toppings.

Leftovers can be stored in an airtight container in the fridge for up to 3 days or frozen for 3 months.

Tips: You can substitute the tofu with chicken, cut into bite-sized pieces.

When you reheat the leftovers in a frying pan, crack an egg over the top and scramble into the rice for a delicious breakfast or snack.

Mince the ginger and garlic in large batches in the food processor or Vitamix and freeze in portions. You will need approximately 90 g (3 oz) of ginger and garlic per portion. Alternatively, buy in a jar. While fresh ginger and garlic will always be our first choice, we understand the importance of convenience in those early postpartum days. Just avoid any with preservatives.

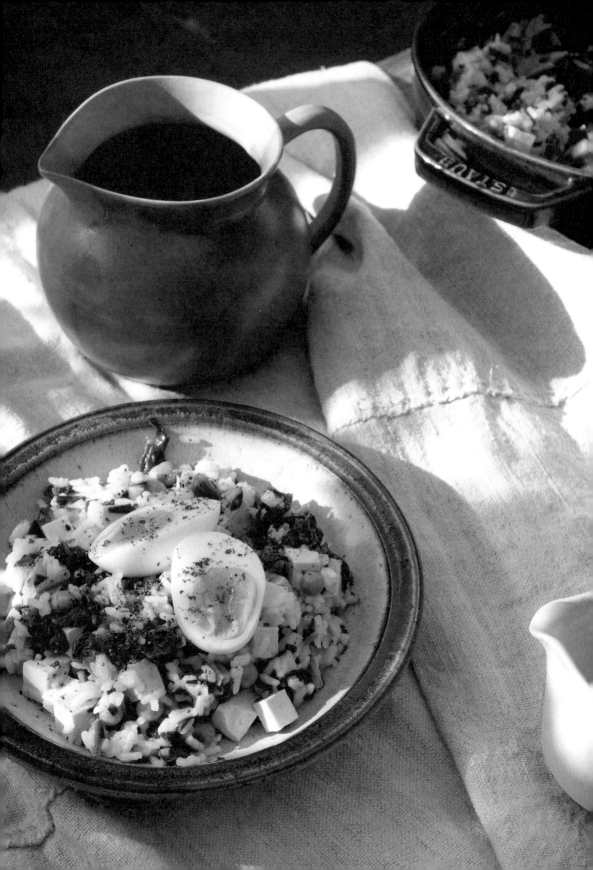

MUSHROOM AND KALE RISOTTO

SERVES 4–6

generous glug of olive oil

100 g (3½ oz) fresh shiitake
  mushrooms, thinly sliced

400 g (14 oz) button
  mushrooms, thinly sliced

large pinch of salt

2 litres (68 fl oz/8 cups)
  vegetable stock or chicken
  broth

1 onion, diced

4 garlic cloves, minced

660 g (1 lb 7 oz/3 cups) arborio
  rice

500 ml (7 fl oz/2 cups) boiling
  water

1 teaspoon dried thyme

½ teaspoon nutmeg

zest and juice of 1 lemon

150 g (5½ oz) fresh or frozen
  kale, shredded

handful of basil leaves, thinly
  sliced (optional)

50 g (1¾ oz) parmesan plus
  extra, to serve, or 25 g
  (½ cup) nutritional yeast

This delicious and moreish meal is packed with immune-boosting shiitake mushrooms and calcium-rich greens. We frequently make this for our postpartum clients who gobble it up in a heartbeat and always request seconds.

Heat the olive oil in a large frying pan over a medium–high heat. Add the mushrooms and a generous pinch of salt, and cook for about 10 minutes, or until the liquid has evaporated and the mushrooms begin to caramelise.

Gently heat the stock in a saucepan.

Meanwhile, heat another generous glug of olive oil in a large pot over a medium heat. Add the onion and cook for 5 minutes. Add the garlic and stir for 2 minutes, or until fragrant then add the rice and stir constantly for approximately one minute, until the rice is translucent.

Add enough stock to just cover the rice and cook, stirring often, until the stock is absorbed. Repeat, adding the remaining stock in increments, until it's all absorbed. Repeat with the water. After approximately 25 minutes the rice should be cooked and creamy.

Add the thyme, nutmeg, lemon zest and juice, cooked mushrooms, shredded kale, and basil, if using, to the rice and stir for about 3–5 minutes, or until the kale is wilted. Add the parmesan plus salt and pepper to taste.

To serve, spoon into bowls and top with additional parmesan or nutritional yeast. Toasted pine nuts also make for a real treat.

Tip: This dish will store in the fridge for up to 3 days or freeze for up to 3 months.

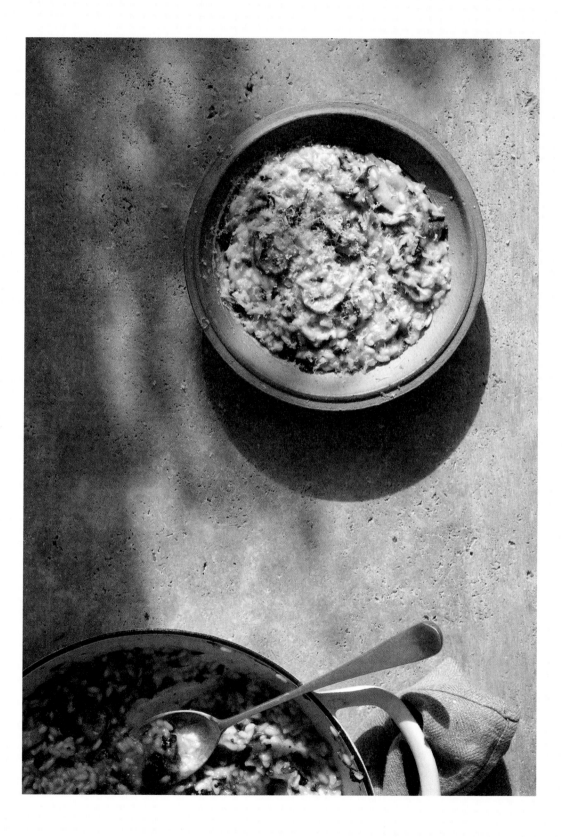

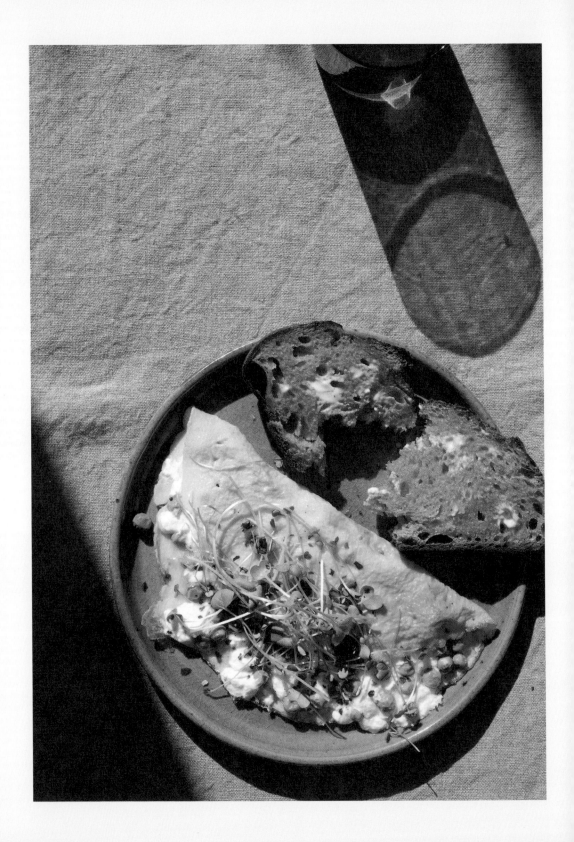

PEA AND GOAT'S FETA OMELETTE

SERVES 1

50 g (1¾ oz/⅓ cup) frozen peas
2 eggs
¼ teaspoon salt
1 teaspoon coconut oil or ghee
1–2 tablespoons goat's feta

To serve (optional):
microherbs
chilli flakes
salad
toasted sourdough

We are definitely not reinventing the wheel by suggesting you make an omelette for breakfast, but we did want to take a moment to remind you that a greens-filled omelette with a piece of wholegrain or sourdough toast makes for a perfectly substantial dinner as well.

We also wanted to take a moment to remind you just how nutritionally dense eggs are. Their whites are packed with protein and their yolks contain vitamins A, D, E and K, plus omega-3, choline and amino acids, making them deeply satiating to a new mama's depleted body while fuelling your body and brain.

Goat's cheese and peas add extra protein to keep you full for hours, but you can and should go wild with different combinations of ingredients. Cooked mushrooms or asparagus, rocket (arugula), corn, salmon, roasted veggies, microherbs and ricotta are some other favourite omelette inclusions in our homes, and you can add chopped herbs to your egg mix if you're feeling fancy.

Pour boiling water over the peas and allow to defrost for 5 minutes while you prepare the other ingredients.

Crack the eggs into a cup, bowl or jug. Add the salt and a tablespoon of water and beat until well combined.

Heat the coconut oil in a frying pan over a medium heat and swirl until it covers the bottom of the pan.

Pour the egg mixture into the pan, swirl until it covers the entire base of the pan and cook for 1 minute.

Drain the peas and add them, with the feta, to one half of the omelette. Cook until the egg is almost firm then gently lift and fold the unfilled half over the filled side.

Continue to cook for another minute or two, then slide onto a plate.

To serve, top with microherbs and chilli flakes or enjoy as is, with a salad or a slice of toasted sourdough.

EGGS AND GREENS

SERVES 1

1 teaspoon coconut oil
150 g (5½ oz) kale, stalks
    removed, washed, leaves cut
    into bite-sized strips
½ teaspoon salt
2 eggs
1 tablespoon kimchi, to serve
Sesame Seaweed Sprinkles
    (p. 229), to taste

If you haven't noticed by now, we love our greens. This quick and easy meal for one is a filling way to get your daily fix with minimal mess and maximum satisfaction.

It may look basic, but these are the kinds of meals you will come back to time and time again, due to their sheer ease, even with a babe in arms. Meals like this are also great for people who are less confident in the kitchen, but want to fuel up with nutritious foods.

Heat the coconut oil in a large frying pan over a medium heat. Add the kale to the pan with the salt and cook for 5 minutes, tossing frequently, until the kale is wilted and starting to brown.

Crack the eggs over the kale and cook for 2–3 minutes, then flip. Cook the eggs for another 2–3 minutes, until the whites are done to your liking. Season with salt and pepper.

Transfer to a bowl and top with kimchi and Sesame Seaweed Sprinkles, plus any other condiments you want to add.

Tip: You can bulk up this meal by popping it in a wrap smeared with hummus and topped with avocado, or keep it simple by serving straight from the pan, with a slice of fresh sourdough.

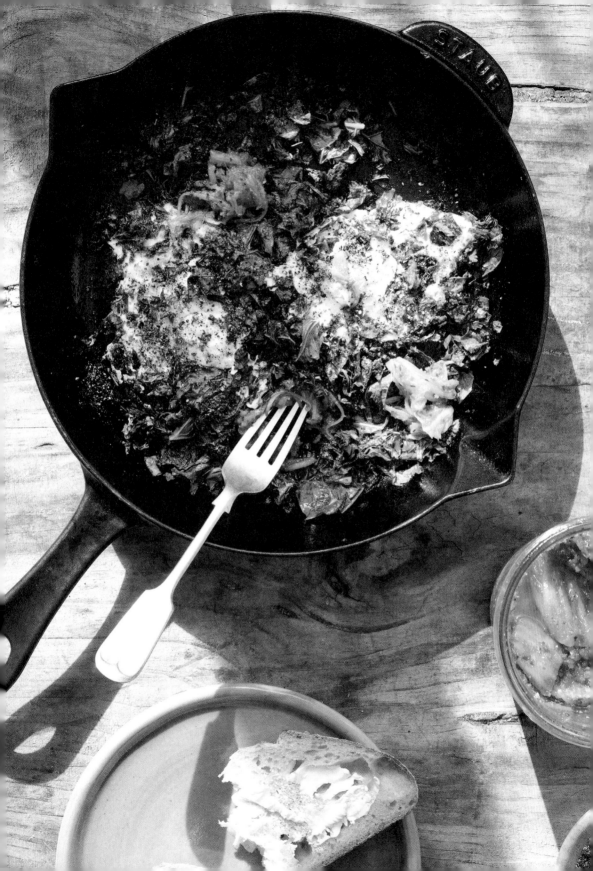

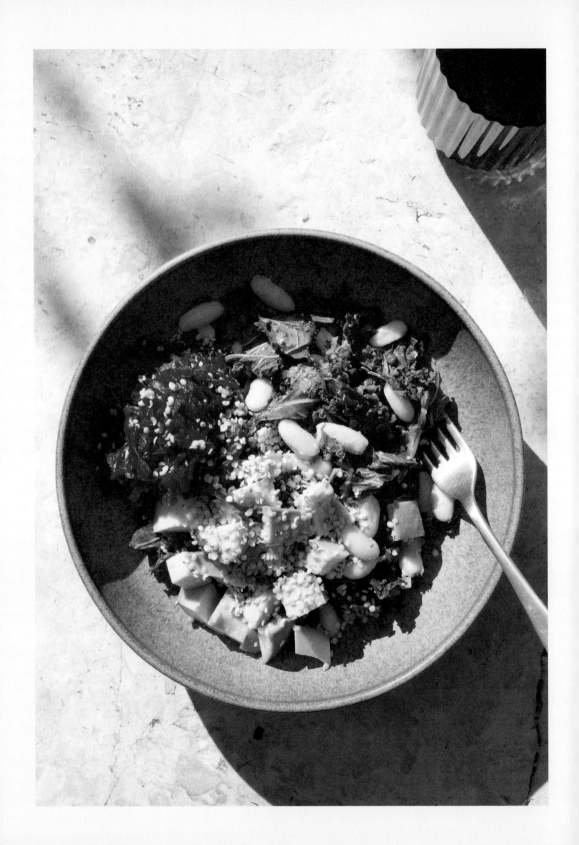

GARLICKY GREENS AND BEANS

SERVES 1–2

1 teaspoon coconut oil

½ bunch of kale, stalks removed, washed, leaves stripped into bite-sized pieces

pinch of salt

400 g (14 oz) tinned cannellini beans, drained and rinsed

juice of ½ lemon

1 garlic clove, minced (or you can microplane it straight into the pan)

To serve:

½ avocado, diced

sauerkraut

1 tablespoon hemp seeds

For those of you who don't love eggs, this is another quick and easy meal for a very hungry person. Ready in less than 5 minutes, it keeps you full for hours, which is important when you are breastfeeding or chasing after an energetic toddler. This makes a lot, so if you are unable to finish it in one sitting, pop the rest aside to graze on as the day goes by, or share with someone in your family. As your babe gets older, they will love eating the beans, avocado and sauerkraut.

Heat the coconut oil in a large frying pan over a medium–high heat. Add the kale (it will look like a lot at first, but will reduce to virtually nothing when cooked, so don't be alarmed!) and a pinch of salt, and sauté for a couple of minutes – then add beans, a squeeze of lemon and the garlic. Toss it all around until the beans are warm and garlic is fragrant, then transfer to a bowl. Top with avo, sauerkraut, hemp seeds and any other herbs/chilli oil you wish to add, along with salt and black pepper to taste.

Tips: Swap kale for baby spinach or frozen spinach if you are in that phase of motherhood where washing and chopping greens is impossible. Nuke frozen spinach in the microwave first, to speed up cooking time.

As with our Eggs and Greens recipe, you can bulk up this meal by popping it in a wrap smeared with hummus or avo or both.

GREENS PIE

SERVES 4–8

150 g (5½ oz/4 cups tightly
   packed) silverbeet (Swiss
   chard), stems removed
150 g (5½ oz/4 cups tightly
   packed) kale, stems removed
100 g (3½ oz/⅔ cup) frozen peas
olive oil for cooking
1 red onion, diced
½ teaspoon sea salt
6–8 garlic cloves, minced
6 large eggs
250 g (9 oz/1 cup) ricotta
¼ teaspoon nutmeg
375 g (13 oz) wholemeal spelt
   pastry or the best quality
   pastry you can find

*Most doulas have a greens pie in their repertoire and for good reason – greens are
some of the most nutrient-dense foods and, when combined with the protein-packed
goodness of eggs and ricotta, provide the perfect fuel for motherhood.*

*When shopping for pastry, look for one that uses butter or olive oil as opposed
to refined vegetable oils, which are high in trans fats and are inflammatory. Where
possible, organic spelt pastry that's made with butter is your best bet.*

Preheat the oven to 210°C (410°F).

Chop the greens into bite-sized pieces. Place in a large bowl and cover with water.
Agitate a little and then allow to sit for a few minutes. Transfer the greens to a colander
in handfuls, shaking as you go so any dirt or sediment stays in the bowl. Rinse the bowl,
add the peas and cover with hot water.

Heat a generous glug of the olive oil in a large frying pan. Add the onion and a pinch
of the salt. Cook for about 5 minutes, stirring regularly, until starting to brown. Add half
the greens and continue stirring regularly for another 5 minutes, or until wilted.

Make a well in the middle. Add another glug of olive oil to the well, add the garlic and
another pinch of the salt and stir within the well constantly for about a minute before
adding the remaining greens and another pinch of salt. Continue stirring regularly
for about another 5 minutes until the greens are cooked. Do a taste test – the greens
should be so tasty that you would happily eat them as is.

Beat the eggs, ricotta and nutmeg in a large mixing bowl with a pinch of salt. Drain the
peas then add, along with the cooled cooked greens. Stir to combine.

Line a pie dish with one sheet of the pastry. Pour the filling in and create a lattice top
with the remaining pastry.

Bake in the preheated oven for 45 minutes. Insert a skewer to check if the egg is cooked
through, then allow to cool for 10 to 15 minutes before slicing and devouring.

Best served warm or at room temperature.

> **Tip:** Leftovers can be stored in the fridge for up to 3 days or in the freezer
> for up to 3 months.

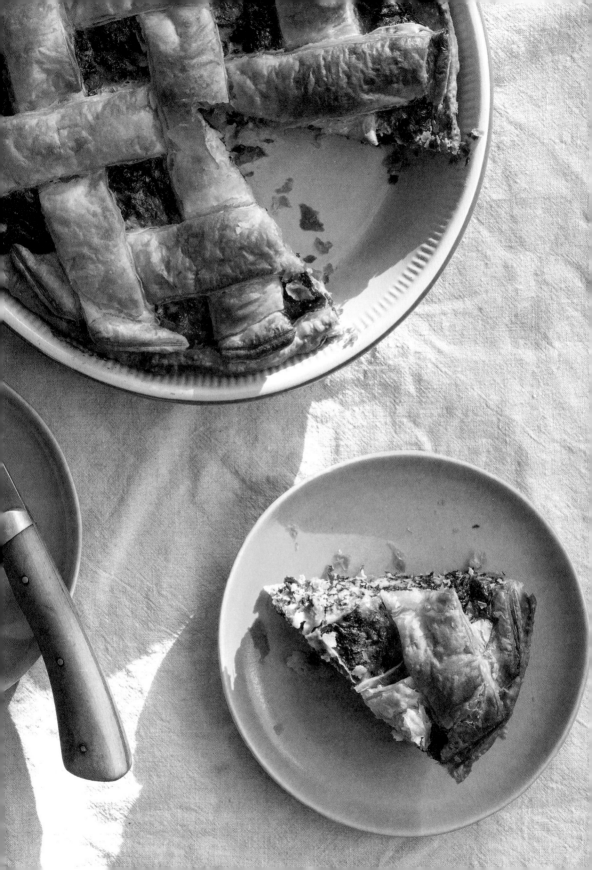

WARM HUG PIE

SERVES 4–6

For the filling:

10 g (¼ oz) porcini mushrooms, blitzed into a chunky powder

olive oil for cooking

1 red onion, diced

3 celery stalks, diced

2 carrots (approx. 500 g/
   1 lb 2 oz), diced

6–8 garlic cloves, minced

2–3 sprigs rosemary

1 heaped teaspoon ground
   coriander

1 heaped teaspoon fennel seeds

1 teaspoon salt

2 tablespoons white-wine
   vinegar

220 g (8 oz) black beluga or
   French green lentils, soaked
   overnight or in boiling water
   for at least one hour

60 g (2 oz/¼ cup) tomato paste
   (concentrated purée)

400 g (14 oz) tinned chickpeas

1 teaspoon sugar

1 teaspoon smoked paprika

250 g (9 oz) frozen spinach

For the topping:

1 head cauliflower, cut into
   bite-sized florets

80 g (2¾ oz/½ cup) cashew nuts

2 tablespoons olive oil or melted
   butter

3 tablespoons nutritional yeast

½ teaspoon sea salt

pinch of nutmeg

Comfort food at its finest, this pie feels like a warm hug from an old friend. The combination of porcini mushrooms, paprika and spices is next-level delicious, and from a naturopathic point of view this dish ticks all the boxes when it comes to protein, fibre, healthy fats, complex carbohydrates, iron, folate, calcium and a variety of prebiotics.

The idea to top this pie with cauliflower came from one of our favourite wholefoods writers Amy Chaplin. Cauliflower is an excellent postpartum food as it supports liver health and the body's ability to process excess hormones.

Soak the porcini mushrooms in 625 ml (21 fl oz/2½ cups) boiling water and set aside.

Heat a generous glug of olive oil in a large pot over a medium heat. Add onion and cook for 5–10 minutes, until starting to brown. Add celery and carrot and continue to cook for another 10 minutes, until softened. If they start to stick at any stage, add a splash of water.

Add garlic, rosemary, coriander, fennel and salt, and cook, stirring constantly, until garlic is fragrant and softened. Add vinegar and give everything a really good stir.

Drain the lentils and add to the pot, along with the porcini mushrooms and their soaking liquid (if you were unable to blitz them before soaking, remove from liquid and finely chop before adding into pot). Cover and cook for 15 minutes, until the lentils are tender.

Stir the tomato paste through the cooked lentils, along with the chickpeas, sugar, smoked paprika and spinach. Cook, stirring often, until the spinach is defrosted and all of its liquid has evaporated.

Season with additional salt and black pepper to taste, then spoon into a pie dish and set aside to cool.

While the filling is cooling, preheat the oven to 200°C (390°F) and get started on the topping.

Place the cauliflower in a steamer (or a colander set over a large pot with a small amount of boiling water in the bottom) and steam for 20–30 minutes, until fork tender.

Transfer to a high-powered blender, along with the remaining topping ingredients and 125 ml (4 fl oz/½ cup) water. Blitz until smooth, scraping bits down from the side if you need.

Pour over the pie filling and smooth with the back of a spoon. Bake for half an hour, or until the top is just starting to brown.

> **Tip:** Soak the cashew nuts in water overnight if you don't have a high-powered blender. Swap for a classic mash if you don't have a blender at all.

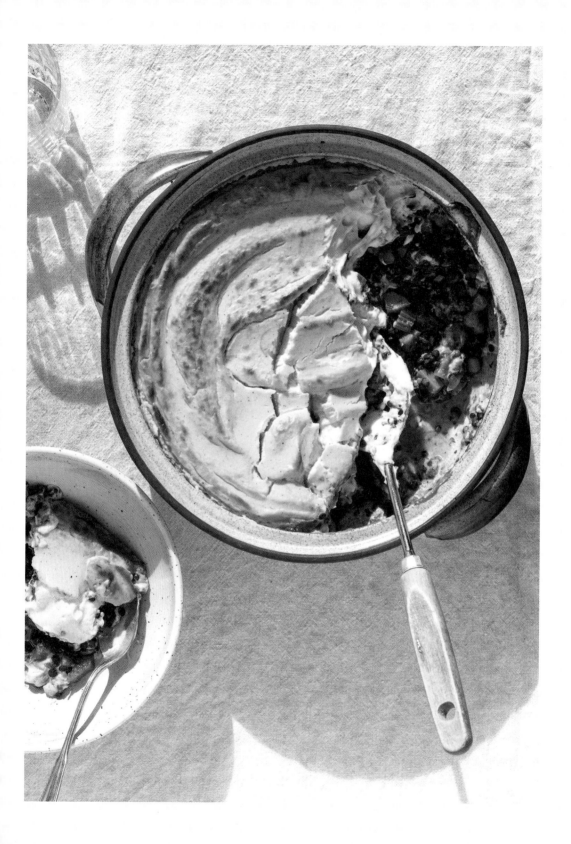

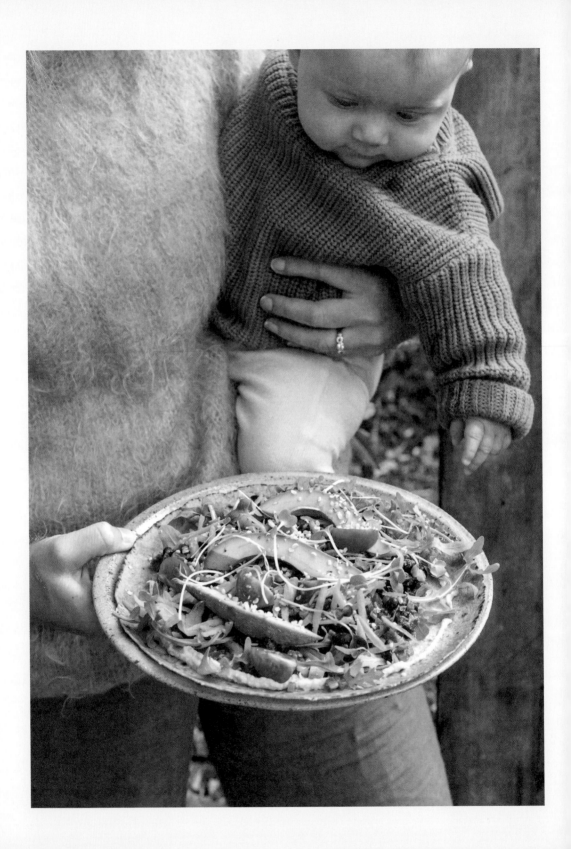

WRAP IT UP

SERVES 2

drizzle of olive oil
1 small red onion, chopped
2 garlic cloves, minced
1 teaspoon ground cumin
1 teaspoon ground coriander
400 g (14 oz) tinned black
    beans, drained and rinsed (or
    1½ cups cooked black beans)
1 teaspoon smoked paprika
½ teaspoon sea salt
2 wholegrain, seeded or gluten-
    free wraps
2 tablespoons hummus or tahini
2 handfuls rocket (arugula) or
    baby spinach
1 carrot, grated
handful of cherry tomatoes,
    diced
1 avocado, sliced
microgreens or coriander
    (cilantro) leaves, to garnish
    (optional)
chilli flakes or hot sauce, to
    taste (optional)

Wraps are great because you can load them with infinitely more nutritious filling than you could ever fit between two slices of bread.

The ingredients we've suggest here are a favourite combo of ours, but you can really go wild with wraps. Instead of hummus or tahini, you can melt cheese onto your wrap when heating it. You can use grated beets instead of carrot; finely sliced red cabbage instead of leafy greens; cannellini beans, minced chicken, or minced beef instead of black beans; and sun-dried tomatoes instead of fresh ones. You could even skip the cooking step altogether and add a tin of tuna instead. Find a combo you love, and enjoy the heck out of it. Your mind and body will thank you.

Heat the oil in a frying pan over a medium–high heat. Add the onion and cook for 5 minutes. Add the garlic, cumin and coriander and stir for a minute or two, until fragrant.

Add the black beans, 60 ml (2 fl oz/¼ cup) water, smoked paprika and salt. Mash the beans a little and give everything a good stir so the water mixes with the beans and you have a creamy, chunky mash. Cook for a couple of minutes until the beans are heated through, then remove from the heat.

Heat the wraps on the stove or in a microwave. Spread a tablespoon of hummus or tahini onto each and fill with the greens, beans, carrot, tomato, avocado and herbs. Add chilli if using. Fold and devour!

Tip: It's important to read the ingredient list when choosing wraps, as many are made using refined vegetable oils, emulsifiers, additives, gums and preservatives, which you want to avoid. Opt for wholemeal or gluten-free options where possible, as these are more nutritious than those made with refined flour.

BUILD YOUR OWN NOURISH BOWL

There is nothing simpler than throwing together a Nourish Bowl. Aim to have one flavour combo per week, and set aside the time to prep about four days' worth of ingredients every Sunday, so that lunch or dinner is taken care of for at least the first half of the week. Lean into the simplicity of eating the same thing multiple days in a row, and relish in the joy of experimentation, finding new favourite flavour combos, trying different grains, and using up stray veggies that are lurking in your fridge.

By making sure you pick one of each thing from the list below, you'll be fuelling your day with complex carbohydrates, balancing your blood sugar with the all-important protein, and helping to regulate your energy and mood with healthy fats.

Start with the base	1–2 cups quinoa, brown rice or other cooked grain of your choice.
Add something green	Such as a handful of sautéed kale, rocket or baby spinach.
Veg it up	Add roasted vegetables like sweet potato, pumpkin, cauliflower, beetroot (beets) or carrot. **Tip:** Roast your vegetables covered in olive or coconut oil and season with your favourite spices or herbs. We always reach for cumin and a generous pinch of sea salt.
Something creamy	We like to use a large dollop of something like hummus, guacamole, pesto or our Green Goodness Dip (overleaf).
Time for protein	Add a chunky protein such as eggs, baked salmon, shredded chicken, spiced ground beef, tempeh, goat's cheese, warmed lentils or beans.
Healthy fats	We love avocado, whole-egg mayonnaise, a drizzle of tahini or a glug of olive oil.
Pickles	Add something fermented and tangy such as sauerkraut, pickled vegetables or kimchi.
Season	Sprinkle with your favourite nuts and seeds. We love sesame seeds, pepitas (pumpkin seeds) and hemp seeds, and we never say no to roasted almonds.
Make it extra special	Add kelp flakes or our Sesame Seaweed Sprinkles (overleaf) (both are great sources of iodine), chilli flakes, olives, dukkah, tzatziki, chutney, lemon juice, coriander or parsley leaves. The world is your oyster, baby!

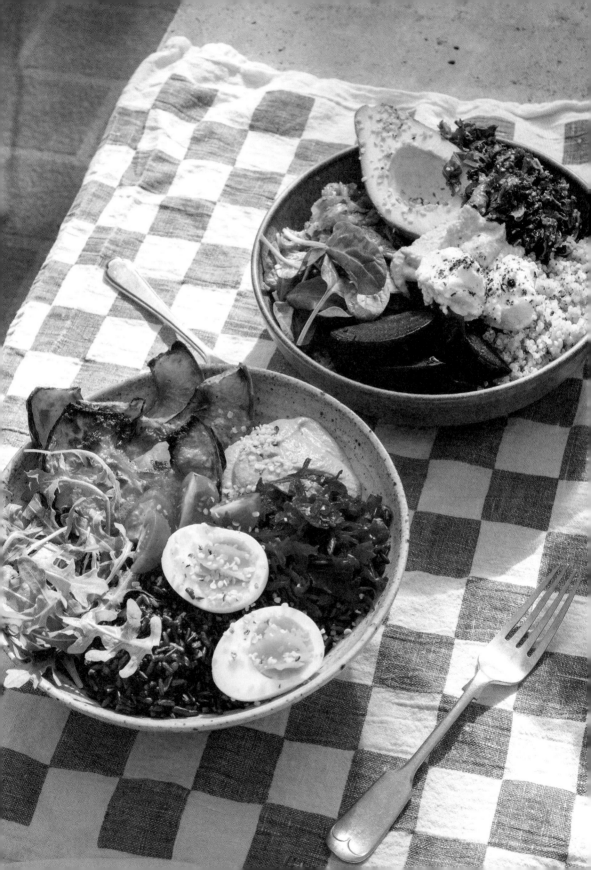

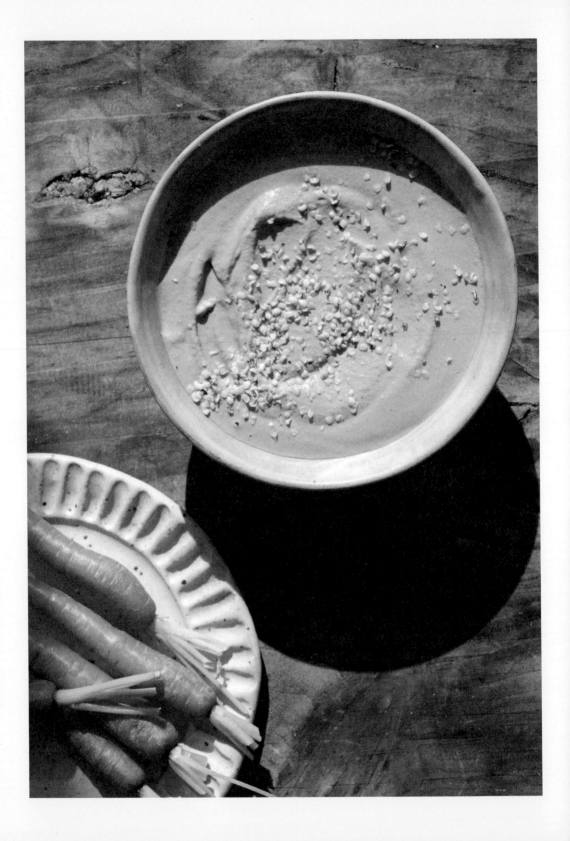

GREEN GOODNESS DIP

This zingy dip is full of nutritious goodness from mineral rich herbs, healthy fats and plant-based protein from hemp seeds and cashews, making it the perfect addition to salads, grilled meat and vegetables, or enjoyed as a healthy snack with crudités. Make it fresh and seasonal by adding whatever herbs you have in the fridge or growing in the garden.

150 g (5½ oz) raw cashew nuts
50 g (1¾ oz/1 cup) basil
20 g (¾ oz/1 cup) parsley
1 tablespoon capers
1 tablespoon sultanas or 1 Medjool date, pitted
1 tablespoon hemp seeds
1½ tablespoons apple-cider vinegar
1 garlic clove
½ teaspoon salt

Place everything in a high-powered blender with 250 ml (8½ fl oz/1 cup) water and blitz until smooth and creamy. Store in an airtight jar in the fridge for up to 5 days.

Delicious on a nourish bowl, smeared on your toast, dolloped on an omelette, dunked with some veggie sticks or stirred into your favourite pasta.

SESAME SEAWEED SPRINKLES

We sprinkle this umami flavour bomb on everything, from avocado loaded sourdough at breakfast to a steaming bowl of noodles at dinnertime. Sea vegetables, including nori, contain iodine, which is essential for healthy thyroid function and metabolism. Good quality sea salt is an abundant source of trace minerals, while the addition of sesame seeds adds a pop of nutty flavour and source of calcium and healthy fats. The perfect postpartum condiment.

10 g (¼ oz) toasted nori flakes
100 g (3½ oz/⅔ cup) toasted black sesame seeds
1 tablespoon sea salt

Place everything in a high-powered blender and blitz for 5–10 seconds, until seaweed is finely chopped and everything is well combined. Store in an airtight jar and sprinkle on literally everything.

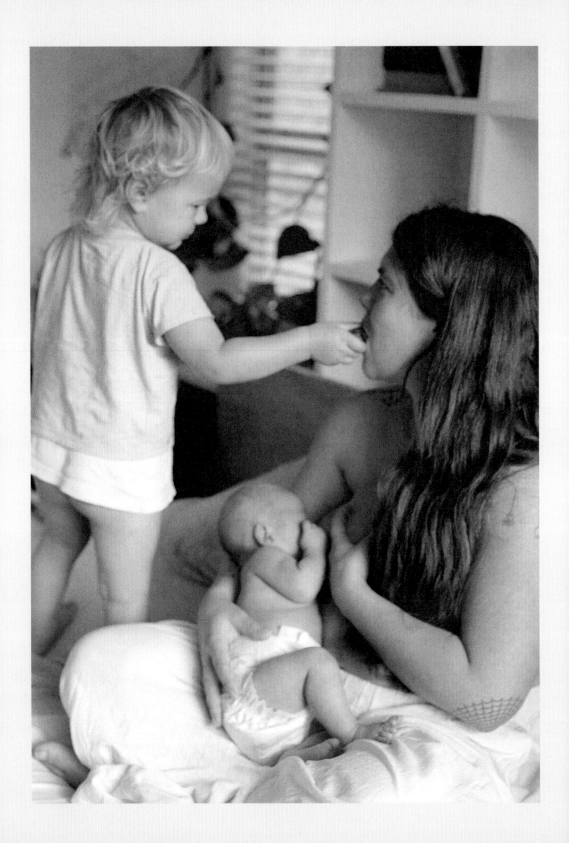

SNACK IDEAS

Make a list of your favourite snacks and meals, and pop it on the fridge so your support people know what to feed you when the 'hanger' sets in. Here are some easy and nutritious options:

- Crackers with hummus, avocado and sprouts
- Dates stuffed with nut butter and topped with hemp seeds
- Wrap filled with hummus, grated carrot, rocket, avocado
- Avocado wrapped in nori sheets
- Veggie sticks with hummus, guacamole or baba ghanoush
- Nuts, chopped apricots and dark chocolate pieces
- Green Goodness Dip (page 229) with celery, carrot and cucumber
- Boiled egg topped with Sesame Seaweed Sprinkles (page 229)
- Egg and hummus on wholegrain toast
- Lettuce cups filled with chickpeas, celery, red onion and mashed avocado.

SMOOTHIE IDEAS

A good rule of thumb when making a smoothie is to use 1 cup of fruit and 1 cup of liquid and always add a protein source to stabilise blood sugar and keep you fuller for longer. Where possible, add a handful of greens for an antioxidant and fibre boost.

- Banana, blueberry, spinach, almond milk and almond butter
- Banana, mango, yoghurt and protein powder
- Raspberry, banana, cacao nibs, chia seeds and coconut milk
- Oats, strawberries, protein powder, yoghurt and oat milk
- Pineapple, spinach, avocado, chia seeds and coconut water
- Kiwi fruit, frozen cauliflower, ginger, fresh lime juice, collagen powder, coconut water

> **Tip:** Prepare your favourite combinations in freezer-friendly containers so you can freeze them and throw them in the blender in a pinch.

RESOURCES

POSTPARTUM

Nurturing Your New Life – Heidi Sze
The First Forty Days – Heng Ou,
    Amely Greeven & Marisa Belger
The Fourth Trimester – Kimberly
    Ann Johnson
Golden Month – Jenny Allison
The Postnatal Depletion Cure –
    Dr Oscar Serrallach
Afterwards Postpartum – Tori
    Bowman Johnson
Zen Mamas – Teresa Palmer and
    Sarah Wright Olsen

BREASTFEEDING

Ina May's Guide to Breastfeeding –
    Ina May Gaskin
Boobin' All Day Boobin' All Night:
    A Gentle Approach to Sleep for
    Breastfeeding Families – Meg Nagle
The Breastfeeding Mother's Guide
    to Making More Milk – Diana West
    and Lisa Marasco
breastfeeding.asn.au
possumsonline.com
kinpostpartumservices.com – The
    Weaning Bible course

BABIES

The Discontented Little Baby –
    Dr Pamela Douglas
Safe Infant Sleep – James J. McKenna
The Continuum Concept – Jean
    Liedloff
tinyheartseducation.com
heysleepybaby.com

PSYCHOLOGY AND MENTAL HEALTH

The Dance of Anger – Harriet Lerner
How to Do the Work – Dr Nicole
    LePera
The Body Keeps the Score – Bessel
    van der Kolk M.D.
The Pink Elephants –
    www.pinkelephants.org.au
SANDS – www.sands.org.au

RELATIONSHIPS

Mating in Captivity – Esther Perel
Rekindling – Dr Martien Snellen
Slow Pleasure – Euphemia Russell

PARENTING

The Montessori Toddler – Simone
    Davies
No Bad Kids – Janet Lansbury
Milk to Meals – Luka McCabe & Carley
    Mendes
boobtofood.com
kidseatincolor.com
7daysofplay.com
biglittlefeelings.com

COOKING

Vegan One-Pot Wonders – Jessica
    Prescott
Village for Mama – Leila Armour

WOMEN'S HEALTH

Period Power – Maisie Hill
In the Flo – Alisa Vitti
The Fifth Vital Sign – Lisa
    Hendrickson-Jack
Period Repair Manual – Lara Briden
Hormone Intelligence – Aviva Romm
Botanical Medicine for Women's
    Health – Aviva Romm

PROSE ON PARENTING

The Motherhood – Jamila Rizvi
Sad Mum Lady – Ashe Davenport
Little Labours – Rivka Galchen
The Course of Love – Alain de Botton
Early Motherhood Poetry & Prose
    Collection – Jessica Urlichs

PODCASTS

The Science of Motherhood
Where Should We Begin? With
    Esther Perel
Tales from the Fourth Trimester
Mother/Other
The Nurtured Village Podcast
Period Power with Maisie Hill
Sex Birth Trauma with Kimberly
    Ann Johnson
Beyond the Bump
Respectful Parenting: Janet Lansbury
    Unruffled
On Being with Krista Tippett
Hidden Brain
Huberman Lab
Newborn Mothers Podcast
The Little Yarrow Podcast
Authentic Sex with Juliet Allen
Australian Birth Stories

AUTHOR BIOS

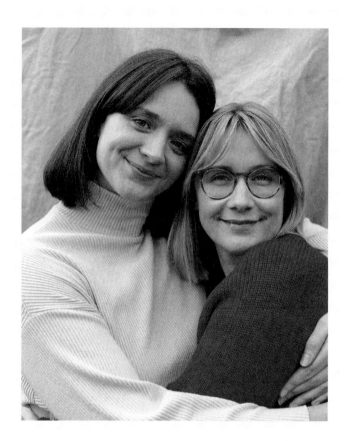

Vaughne is a qualified naturopath and full-spectrum doula with a dedication to educating and supporting women and families from preconception to the postpartum and beyond. Jess is a mother of two, cookbook author and postpartum doula. She has written three books with Hardie Grant London: *Vegan Goodness, Vegan Goodness Feasts* and *Vegan One-Pot Wonders*.

In 2019, Vaughne and Jess launched their business Mama Goodness, which creates nourishing comfort food and botanical products to support people through all phases of motherhood. Their days are filled with endless conversations about mothers, the struggles new parents face, nutrition and all the ways in which they wish they could help; this book is their contribution.

ACKNOWLEDGEMENTS

Our mothers, postpartum clients, and families in our community from whom we have learnt so much.

Andy, Louie and Jude, for your patience and support while this book stole your wife and mama away for extended periods of time.

Alice, for believing in us and making this book a possibility.

Antonietta, for holding our hands the whole way through.

Hannah, Allison, Roxy and Amanda for your editing and proofreading prowess.

Kristin, for your tasteful eye, and Vanessa for your incredible patience while we finessed, finessed and finessed some more.

Lee and Meryl, for making our recipes look more beautiful than we ever possibly could, and for making the recipe shoot days so fun and seamless.

All of our beautiful contributors and models whom we list on page 236.

And last but most certainly not least, our readers. We love you.

REFERENCES

Australian Breastfeeding Association (2017). 'Antenatal expressing of Colostrum.' Retrieved from: https://www.breastfeeding.asn.au/bfinfo/antenatal-expression-colostrum

Badr, H. A. & Zauszniewski, J.A. (2017). Kangaroo care and postpartum depression: The role of oxytocin. *International Journal of Nursing Sciences*, 4(2), 179–183, https://doi.org/10.1016/j.ijnss.2017.01.001.

Bergman, A., Heindel, J. J., Jobling, S., Kidd, K. A., & Zoeller, T. R. (2013). State of the science of endocrine disrupting chemicals 2012: summary for decision-makers. *World Health Organization, United Nations Environment Programme, Inter-Organization Programme for the Sound Management of Chemicals*. Retrieved from: https://apps.who.int/iris/handle/10665/78102

Beyond Blue (2015). 'Healthy Dads.' Retrieved from: https://www.beyondblue.org.au/about-us/about-our-work/our-work-with-men/healthy-dadshttps://www.beyondblue.org.au/docs/default-source/researchproject-files/bw0313-beyondblue-healthy-dads-full-report.pdf?sfvrsn=6f0243ea_0

Bilal, M., Mehmood, S., & Iqbal, H. M. N. (2020). The Beast of Beauty: Environmental and Health Concerns of Toxic Components in Cosmetics. *Cosmetics*, 7(1):13. https://doi.org/10.3390/cosmetics7010013

Bohren, M. A., Hofmeyr, G. J., Sakala, C., Fukuzawa, R. K., & Cuthbert, A. (2017). Continuous support for women during childbirth. The Cochrane database of systematic reviews, 7(7), CD003766. https://doi.org/10.1002/14651858.CD003766.pub6

Burns E. (2014). More than clinical waste? Placenta rituals among Australian home-birthing women *The Journal of perinatal education*, 23(1), 41–49. https://doi.org/10.1891/1058-1243.23.1.41

Centre of Perinatal Excellence (n.d). 'Postnatal Anxiety.' Retrieved from: https://www.cope.org.au/new-parents/postnatal-mental-health-conditions/postnatal-anxiety/

Centre of Perinatal Excellence (n.d). 'Postnatal Depression.' Retrieved from: https://www.cope.org.au/new-parents/postnatal-mental-health-conditions/postnatal-depression/

Chang, C. Y., Ke, D. S., & Chen, J. Y. (2009). Essential fatty acids and the human brain. *Acta neurologica Taiwanica*, 18(4), 231–241.

Chapman, G. D. (2010). *The 5 Love Languages®: The Secret to Love That Lasts*. Walker Large Print.

Chekroud, S. R., Gueorguieva, R., Zheutlin, A. B., Paulus, M., Krumholz, H. M., Krystal, J. H. et al. (2018). Association between physical exercise and mental health in 1·2 million individuals in the USA between 2011 and 2015: a cross-sectional study. *The Lancet Psychiatry*, 5(9), 739–746. https://doi.org/10.1016/S2215-0366(18)30227-X

The Chemical Maze https://chemicalmaze.com/

Dennis, C.-L., Fung, K., Grigoriadis, S., Robinson, G. E., Romans, S., & Ross, L. (2007). Traditional Postpartum Practices and Rituals: A Qualitative Systematic Review. *Women's Health*, 487–502. https://doi.org/10.2217/17455057.3.4.487

DiNicolantonio, J. J., & O'Keefe, J. H. (2018). Importance of maintaining a low omega-6/omega-3 ratio for reducing inflammation. *Open heart*, 5(2), e000946. https://doi.org/10.1136/openhrt-2018-000946

Douglas, P. (2014). *The Discontented Little Baby*. University of Queensland Press.

Endocrine Disruptors (2020). https://www.endocrine.org/-/media/endocrine/files/topics/edc_guide_2020_v1_6chqennew-version.pdf

Environmental Working Group. (2022). Dirty Dozen: EWG's 2022 shoppers guide to pesticides in produce. https://www.ewg.org/foodnews/dirty-dozen.php

EWG's Skin Deep – Safe Skincare Products https://www.ewg.org/skindeep/

Field, T., & Diego, M. (2008). Vagal activity, early growth and emotional development. *Infant behavior & development*, 31(3), 361–373. https://doi.org/10.1016/j.infbeh.2007.12.008

Flaws, J., Damdimopoulou, P., Patisaul, H. B., Gore, A., Raetzman, L., & Vandenberg, L. N. (2020). Plastic, EDCs & Health: A guide for public interest organizations and policy makers on endocrine disrupting chemicals and plastics.

Forman, J., & Silverstein, J. (2012). Organic Foods: Environmental Advantages and Disadvantages. *American Academy of Pediatrics*, 130 (5), 1406–1415. https://doi.org/10.1542/peds.2012-2579

Gridneva, Z., Rea, A., Tie, W. J., Lai, C. T., Kugananthan, S., Ward, L. C., Murray, K., Hartmann, P. E., & Geddes, D. T. (2019). Carbohydrates in Human Milk and Body Composition of Term Infants during the First 12 Months of Lactation. *Nutrients*, 11(7), 1472. https://doi.org/10.3390/nu11071472

Gotman, J (n.d). Retrieved from https://www.gottman.com/blog/turn-toward-instead-of-away/

Hansford, L. (n.d). 'What's the big deal with skin to skin?' Retrieved from: https://www.laleche.org.uk/whats-big-deal-skin-skin/

Hardwicke-Collings, J. (date unknown). Minmia blog series 2: getting the birth ceremony right. Retrieved from: https://janehardwickecollings.com/minmia-blog-series-2-getting-the-birth-ceremony-right/

Harrington, C. T., Al Hafid, N., & Waters, K. A. (2022). Butyrylcholinesterase is a potential biomarker for Sudden Infant Death Syndrome, *eBioMedicine, 80*. https://doi.org/10.1016/j.ebiom.2022.104041.

Hassiotou F, Hepworth AR, Williams TM, Twigger A-J, Perrella S, Lai CT, et al. (2013). Breastmilk Cell and Fat Contents Respond Similarly to Removal of Breastmilk by the Infant. *PLoS ONE 8*(11): e78232. https://doi.org/10.1371/journal.pone.0078232

Health.vic (n.d.). 'Implementing Evidence based practice.' Retrieved from: https://www2.health.vic.gov.au/hospitals-and-health-services/patient-care/older-people/resources/improving-access/ia-evidence

Hoekzema, E., Barba-Müller, E., Pozzobon, C., Picado, M., Lucco, F., García-García, D., Soliva, J. C., Tobeña, A., Desco, M., Crone, E. A., Ballesteros, A., Carmona, S., & Vilarroya, O. (2017). Pregnancy leads to long-lasting changes in human brain structure. *Nature neuroscience, 20*(2), 287–296. https://doi.org/10.1038/nn.4458

Jamieson, D. J., Theiler, R. N., & Rasmussen, S. A. (2006). Emerging infections and pregnancy. *Emerging infectious diseases, 12*(11), 1638–1643. https://doi.org/10.3201/eid1211.060152

Johnson, K. A. (2017). *The Fourth Trimester: A Postpartum Guide to Healing Your Body, Balancing Your Emotions, and Restoring Your Vitality.* Shambahla.

Keikha, M., Shayan-Moghadam, R., Bahreynian, M., & Kelishadi, R. (2021). Nutritional supplements and mother›s milk composition: a systematic review of interventional studies. *International breastfeeding journal, 16*(1), 1. https://doi.org/10.1186/s13006-020-00354-0

Kent, J. C. Mitoulas, L.R. Cregan, M.D. Ramsay, D.T. Doherty, D.A. Hartman, P.E. (2006). Volume and Frequency of Breastfeedings and Fat Content of Breast Milk Throughout the Day. *Pediatrics,* 117(3), e387–e395. https://doi.org/10.1542/Peds.2005-1417

Kim P. (2016). Human Maternal Brain Plasticity: Adaptation to Parenting. *New directions for child and adolescent development, 2016*(153), 47–58. https://doi.org/10.1002/cad.20168

Korsmo, H. W., Jiang, X., & Caudill, M. A. (2019). Choline: Exploring the Growing Science on Its Benefits for Moms and Babies. *Nutrients,* 11(8), 1823. https://doi.org/10.3390/nu11081823

Macpherson, A. J., de Agüero, M. G., & Ganal-Vonarburg, S. C. (2017). How nutrition and the maternal microbiota shape the neonatal immune system. *Nature reviews. Immunology,* 17(8), 508–517. https://doi.org/10.1038/nri.2017.58

Martínez-García, M., Paternina-Die, M., Desco, M., Vilarroya, O., & Carmona, S. (2021). Characterizing the Brain Structural Adaptations Across the Motherhood Transition. *Frontiers in global women's health, 2,* 742775. https://doi.org/10.3389/fgwh.2021.742775

Mead M. N. (2008). Benefits of sunlight: a bright spot for human health. *Environmental health perspectives,* 116(4), A160–A167. https://doi.org/10.1289/ehp.116-a160

The Milk Meg. (2019). Conflicting Breastfeeding Advice: Who should I listen to? Retrieved from: https://themilkmeg.com/conflicting-breastfeeding-advice-whoshould-i-listen-to/

Moberg, K. U., Handlin, L., & Petersson, M. (2020). Neuroendocrine mechanisms involved in the physiological effects caused by skin-to-skin contact – With a particular focus on the oxytocinergic system, *Infant Behavior and Development, 61.* https://doi.org/10.1016/j.infbeh.2020.101482

Nourmoradi, H., Foroghi, M., Farhadkhani, M., & Vahid Dastjerdi, M. (2013). Assessment of lead and cadmium levels in frequently used cosmetic products in Iran. *Journal of environmental and public health,* 2013, 962727. https://doi.org/10.1155/2013/962727

Olff, M., Frijling, J. L., Kubzansky, L. D., Bradley, B., Ellenbogen, M. A., Cardoso, C., Bartz, J. A., Yee, J. R., & van Zuiden, M. (2013). The role of oxytocin in social bonding, stress regulation and mental health: An update on the moderating effects of context and interindividual differences. *Psychoneuroendocrinology,* 38(9), 1883–1894. https://doi.org/10.1016/j.psyneuen.2013.06.019

Patterson, E., Wall, R., Fitzgerald, G. F., Ross, R. P., & Stanton, C. (2012). Health implications of high dietary omega-6 polyunsaturated Fatty acids. *Journal of nutrition and metabolism,* 2012, 539426. https://doi.org/10.1155/2012/539426

Pickett, E. (2011). The Dangerous Game of the Feeding Interval Obsession. Retrieved from: https://www.emmapickettbreastfeedingsupport.com/twitter-andblog/the dangerous-game-of-the-feeding-interval-obsession

Ramirez, J., Guarner, F., Bustos Fernandez, L., Maruy, A., Sdepanian, V. L., & Cohen, H. (2020). Antibiotics as Major Disruptors of Gut Microbiota. *Frontiers in cellular and infection microbiology,* 10, 572912. https://doi.org/10.3389/fcimb.2020.572912

Rasmussen, B., Ennis, M., Pencharz, P., Ball, R., Courtney-Martin, G., & Elango, R. (2020). Protein Requirements of Healthy Lactating Women Are Higher Than the Current Recommendations. *Current Developments in Nutrition, 4*(2), 653. https://doi.org/10.1093/cdn/nzaa049_046

Restorative Rest – Huberman https://www.youtube.com/watch?v=nm1TxQj9IsQ&ab_ channel=AndrewHuberman

Riley, M. (2022). *The First Year of Parenthood: New Parents and Their Sleep Patterns.* Retrieved from The Sleep Junkie: https://www.sleepjunkie.com/new-parents-and-sleep/

Serrallach, O. (2018). 'The Goop: Are you still recovering from pregnancy years later?' Retrieved from Apple Podcasts.

Serrallach, O. (2018). *The Postnatal Depletion Cure: A Complete Guide to Rebuilding Your Health and Restoring Your Energy for Mothers of Newborns, Toddlers, and Young Children.* Grand Central Publishing.

Shannon, S., Lewis, N., Lee, H., & Hughes, S. (2019). Cannabidiol in Anxiety and Sleep: A Large Case Series. *The Permanente journal,* 23, 18–041. https://doi.org/10.7812/TPP/18-041

Simpson, J. L., Bailey, L. B., Pietrzik, K., Shane, B., & Holzgreve, W. (2010). Micronutrients and women of reproductive potential: required dietary intake and consequences of dietary deficiency or excess. Part I–Folate, Vitamin B12, Vitamin B6. *The journal of maternal-fetal & neonatal medicine: the official journal of the European Association of Perinatal Medicine, the Federation of Asia and Oceania Perinatal Societies, the International Society of Perinatal Obstetricians,* 23(12), 1323–1343. https://doi.org/10.3109/14767051003678234

Stanford University. (2020). 'Breastfeeding: Hand expression of breastmilk.' Retrieved from: https://med.stanford.edu/newborns/professional-education/breastfeeding/handexpressing-Milk.html

Taft, A. J., Shankar, M., Black, K. I., Mazza, D., Hussainy, S., & Lucke, J. C. (2018). Unintended and unwanted pregnancy in Australia: a cross-sectional, national random telephone survey of prevalence and outcomes. *The Medical Journal of Australia*, 209(9), 407–408. https://doi.org/10.5694/mja17.01094

Tähkämö, L., Partonen, T., & Pesonen, A. K. (2019). Systematic review of light exposure impact on human circadian rhythm. *Chronobiology international*, 36(2), 151–170. https://doi.org/10.1080/07420528.2018.1527773

Thomas, P. A., & Kim, S. (2021). Lost Touch? Implications of Physical Touch for Physical Health. The journals of gerontology. *Series B, Psychological sciences and social* sciences, 76(3), e111–e115. https://doi.org/10.1093/geronb/gbaa134

Thurston, R. C., Luther, J. F., Wisniewski, S. R., Eng, H., & Wisner, K. L. (2013). Prospective evaluation of nighttime hot flashes during pregnancy and postpartum. *Fertility and sterility, 100*(6), 1667–1672. https://doi.org/10.1016/j.fertnstert.2013.08.020

Trickey, Ruth. (2011). Women, hormones & the menstrual cycle. Fairfield, Vic: Melbourne Holistic Health Group

UNICEF (n.d) BFHI Resources. 'Skin-to-skin contact.' Retrieved from: https://www.unicef.org.uk/babyfriendly/baby-friendly-resources/implementingstandards-resources/skin-to-skin-contact/

Vaglio, S. (2009). Chemical communication and mother-infant recognition. *Communicative & integrative biology, 2*(3), 279–281. https://doi.org/10.4161/cib.2.3.8227

Vitti, A. (2021). Infradian Rhythm: Your Guide to a Perfect Cycle. *Flo Living*. Retrieved from: https://www.floliving.com/infradian-rhythm/

Wastyk, H. C., Fragiadakis, G. K., Perelman, D., Dahan, D., Merrill, B. D., Yu, F. B., Topf, M., Gonzalez, C. G., Van Treuren, W., Han, S., Robinson, J. L., Elias, J. E., Sonnenburg, E. D., Gardner, C. D., & Sonnenburg, J. L. (2021). Gut-microbiota-targeted diets modulate human immune status. *Cell, 184*(16), 4137–4153.e14. https://doi.org/10.1016/j.cell.2021.06.019

CONTRIBUTORS & COLLABORATORS

- Renee White
- Amy Sherer
- Aimee Anderson
- Catie Gett
- Lilly Lowrey
- Hannah Clark
- Kaitlin Bywater
- Dr Sophie Brock
- Euphemia Russell

MODELS

- Sonia Gill and Ilya Lee
- Rangi and Amrith De Silva
- Raffaella Kaiser Grove, Alva and Zsa Zsa Kaiser Johnson, Will Johnson
- Nina Lake and Michael Longton
- Carol Onopaka Yema and Sylvia Mado Makonda
- Alice and Billie Hardie-Grant
- Roberta Nelson and Sophia Nelson-Marks
- Yahna Fookes and Sunday Kucyk
- Laura and Archie Bloom
- Leah Harris and Rosie Challinor
- Cat Webb and August Webb Kerr
- Sara Watts and Laurence Huxley Watts
- Claire, Hannah and Goldie Eden
- Anna, Bec and Quinn McLay
- Tania Rahman and Eztli Rahman Kirk
- Elise Brain, Toby and Frank Mackisack
- Andrew Ketteridge, Louie Ketteridge, Jude Ketteridge

INDEX

Note: this index covers topics and themes in the book. For a list of recipes refer to page 177.

CREDITS

Excerpt from *Golden Month* on page 7 © Jenny Allison 2021, reproduced with permission of Beatnik Publishing.

Excerpt from *Ten Moons* on page 21 © Jane Hardwicke Collings 2016, reproduced with permission.

Excerpt from *The 5 Love Languages®: The Secret to Love That Lasts* on pages 32–33 © Gary Chapman 2015, reproduced with permission of Moody Publishers.

Excerpt from *Nurturing Your New Life* on page 44 © Heidi Sze 2019, reproduced with permission of HarperCollins Publishers Australia Pty Limited.

Excerpt from *The Dangerous Game of the Feeding Interval Obsession* on page 52 © Emma Pickett 2011, reproduced with permission.

Excerpt on page 70 originally printed in *clarity & connection* copyright © 2021 by Diego Perez Lacera, published by Andrews McMeel Publishing, reproduced with permission.

Excerpt from *Commentary: Does 'Cry It Out' Really Have No Adverse Effects on Attachment? Reflections on Bilgin and Wolke* on page 79 © Abi Davis and Robin Kramer 2020, reproduced with permission.

Excerpt from *The Fourth Trimester* on page 85 © Kimberly Ann Johnson 2018, reproduced with permission.

Excerpt on page 129 from *Birth Without Fear* by January Harshe, copyright © 2019. Reprinted by permission of Hachette Books, an imprint of Hachette Book Group, Inc.

Excerpt on page 130 reproduced with permission from *The Postnatal Depletion Cure* by Dr Oscar Serralach, Hachette Australia, 2018.

Excerpt from *Blood Rites* on page 135 © Jane Hardwicke Collings 2022, reproduced with permission.

Excerpt from *The Dangers of 'Crying It Out'* on page 143 © Darcia Navarez, PhD 2011, reproduced with permission.

Excerpt on page 150 © Martien Snellen, from *Rekindling: Your Relationship After Childbirth*, published by The Text Publishing Company, 2010, reproduced with permission.

Excerpt on page 151 from *Mating in Captivity* by Esther Perel. Copyright © 2006 by Esther Perel. Used by permission of HarperCollins Publishers.

Text on pages 170–171 © Dr Sophie Brock 2022, reproduced with permission.

Quote on page 14 © Naomi Chrisoulakis 2021, reproduced with permission.

Quote on page 14 © Christine Devlin Eck, reproduced with permission.

Quote on page 20 © Nikki McMahon 2021, reproduced with permission.

Quote on page 55 © Carley Mendes 2021, reproduced with permission.

Quote on page 71 © Joy Kusek 2013, reproduced with permission.

Quote on page 78 © Aviva Romm 2019, reproduced with permission.

Quote on page 149 © Emily Hehir 2022, reproduced with permission.

Quote on page 149 © Amy Pearson 2022, reproduced with permission.

Quote on page 149 © Rowie Cooke 2022, reproduced with permission.

Quote on page 169 © Daphne Delvaux, Esq. 2021, reproduced with permission.

Published in 2023 by Hardie Grant Books, an imprint of Hardie Grant Publishing

Hardie Grant Books (Melbourne)
Wurundjeri Country
Building 1, 658 Church Street
Richmond, Victoria 3121

Hardie Grant Books (London)
5th & 6th Floors
52–54 Southwark Street
London SE1 1UN

hardiegrant.com/au/books

Hardie Grant acknowledges the Traditional Owners of the country on which we work, the Wurundjeri people of the Kulin nation and the Gadigal people of the Eora nation, and recognises their continuing connection to the land, waters and culture. We pay our respects to their Elders past and present.

All rights reserved. No part of this publication may be reproduced, stored in a retrieval system or transmitted in any form by any means, electronic, mechanical, photocopying, recording or otherwise, without the prior written permission of the publishers and copyright holders.

The moral rights of the authors have been asserted.

Copyright text © Jessica Prescott and Vaughne Geary 2023
Copyright photography © Jessica Prescott 2023
    except page 130 © Tanya Anderson 2023, page 233 © Cara Mand 2023
Copyright design © Hardie Grant Publishing 2023

Every effort has been made to trace, contact and acknowledge all copyright holders. Please contact the publisher with any information on errors or omissions.

A catalogue record for this book is available from the National Library of Australia

Life After Birth
ISBN 978 1 74379 819 5

10 9 8 7 6 5 4 3 2 1

Publisher: Alice Hardie-Grant
Project Editor: Antonietta Melideo
Editor: Hannah Hempenstall
Design Manager: Kristin Thomas
Designer: Vanessa Masci | Studio Terra
Photographer: Jessica Prescott
Stylist: Lee Blaylock
Home Economist: Meryl Batlle
Production Manager: Todd Rechner

Colour reproduction by Splitting Image Colour Studio
Printed in China by Leo Paper Products LTD.

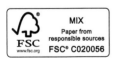

The paper this book is printed on is from FSC®-certified forests and other sources. FSC® promotes environmentally responsible, socially beneficial and economically viable management of the world's forests.